LIVING
PROOF

A Medical Mutiny

MICHAEL GEARIN-TOSH

SCRIBNER
New York London Toronto Sydney Singapore

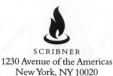

SCRIBNER
1230 Avenue of the Americas
New York, NY 10020

First Scribner U.S. Edition 2002
Published by arrangement with Simon & Schuster UK Ltd.
Originally published in Great Britain in 2002 by Scribner,
an imprint of Simon & Schuster UK Ltd.

SCRIBNER and design are trademarks of Macmillan Library Reference USA, Inc.,
used under license by Simon & Schuster, the publisher of this work.

For information about special discounts for bulk purchases,
please contact Simon & Schuster Special Sales:
1-800-456-6798 or business@simonandschuster.com

Appendix by Dr. Carmen Wheatley for Caliban Scripts Ltd.

Extract from *Raw Energy* by Leslie Kenton published by Vermillion.
Used by permission of the Random House Group Limited.
Before I Say Goodbye, Ruth Picardie.
Reproduced by permission of Penguin Books Ltd.
Life's Too Short, Helen Rollason.
Reproduced by permission of Hodder and Stoughton Limited.
Science and the Quiet Art, Sir David Weatherall.
By permission of Oxford University Press.

DESIGNED BY ERICH HOBBING

Text set in Bembo

Manufactured in the United States of America

3   5   7   9   10   8   6   4   2

Library of Congress Cataloging-in-Publication Data
Gearin-Tosh, Michael
Living proof : a medical mutiny / Michael Gearin-Tosh.—1st ed.
p.   cm.
Includes bibliographical reference.
1. Gearin-Tosh, Michael—Health. 2. Multiple myeloma—Patients—
Great Britain—Biography. 3. Cancer—Alternative treatment
I. Title.
RC280.B6G435   2002
362.1'96994'0092—dc21
[B]   2002017739

ISBN 0-7432-2517-1

CONTENTS

Living Proof

FOREWORD

The diagnosis is cancer.

The hospital tells me to start chemotherapy at once. Without it I will die in months; with it I may live for two to three years.

I ask for a second opinion.

The advice is the same: start at once.

Then a world authority on cancer says that if I touch chemotherapy, I am "a goner."

Which advice do I take? Should I look elsewhere? Do I have time?

The opposite of the phrase *Living Proof* is, I suggest, *dead wrong*.

Or, if you will, wrong and dead.

The stakes are high.

What am I to do?

FOREWORD

1

March

I have no sense of being ill as I leave Oxford, where I teach in the University, for a trip to Moscow. The flight is via Paris, where a Russian lady boards.

She refuses to take her seat.

"But it is by the window, Madame."

"You must change," she tells the stewardess, "it will frighten my dog."

A puppy is in her coat and looks relieved to stay there. But a dog on a plane . . . what a difference from UK quarantine. And in Moscow everyone is out with a pet before going to work.

From the window of the tower block where I stay I can see spaniels, terriers, Samoyeds and a dog like a wolf. The owners smoke and take care on the ice: the only light is from street lamps, which are not bright. Dawn will not come to Moscow for a couple of hours.

My visit is at the invitation of the Russian Academy of Theatre Arts. Founded by the Czar's family in 1878, the Academy continued through the Revolution and still occupies the same building not far from the Kremlin. Where the Royal

Academy of Dramatic Art in London has ninety students on a three-year course, the Russian Academy has five hundred students for five years. Even in my class you sense a different scale: I meet Cossacks, a Tartar, a girl from St. Petersburg who could be a ballerina, Muscovites, students who look Scandinavian and others who come from the regions near China. All twelve time zones of Russia have been crossed to bring us together.

My task is to direct scenes from Shakespeare. As we start a Professor of the Russian Academy walks in. He comes with an entourage of two well-built ladies and a lithe assistant who smokes Turkish.

I am told to stand up.

"What is your positioning with regard to truth?" the Professor asks me.

I answer as best I can, but not well enough.

Am I not concerned, the Professor enquires, with Shakespeare's tendency to fantasy? And what of privilege in the plays?

One of the Professor's ladies writes down what is said, the second keeps an eye on me and the smoker smiles at the Professor.

He now asks me to explain the teaching of drama in the United Kingdom.

I reply that there is no single method, and that each of the British schools has their own emphasis. At the Oxford School of Drama—not a part of the University of Oxford—the philosophy is to spend the first months concentrating on verse not prose.

"Russian students do not open their mouths until they study the throat and larynx," the Professor says.

Not a hint of protest on the faces of the students.

April

"You look pale," says Rachel as she meets me at Heathrow.

"No sun in Moscow."

"Even now?"

"It was bright on a couple of afternoons, for an hour or so. Still cold, but people tried to sunbathe: men took off their shirts and lined up in the streets."

In contrast, there is high spring in the south of England. We sit in our garden at Oxford and listen to a blackbird: in Moscow, there were only crows.

Rachel Trickett and I have lived together for twenty-five years. We are not married, and we are not lovers. If this makes us an odd couple, neither of us gives it a thought. We adore each other's company, and Rachel, daughter of a postman from Wigan, is fierce about her independence and the value of privacy.

We are both scholars of English Literature.

Rachel has retired from her official position as Principal of St. Hugh's College, one of the colleges in the University. But she continues to teach both undergraduate and post-graduate students. She gives lectures to universities in the UK and the States and, at present, she is preparing a number of broadcasts for the BBC.

May

Oxford term starts and our weeks are full of lessons, lectures and the business of University life.

At the end of the month I catch a chill. Nothing to it, we think: I was gardening for too long in the rain. But after a day in bed I wake up wet as if I were swimming. I take off the sheets and wrap myself in towels.

Two hours later, wet again.

Rachel hates doctors—her own tells her to stop smoking and to drink less whisky—but she insists that I take advice.

I phone a doctor, who recommends paracetamol.

Two more sweating nights.

"Keep up the paracetamol," the doctor repeats on the phone "and drink plenty fluids."

After further nights I argue when I ring. "Is not this sweating very unusual?"

"Possibly, but you are fifty-four."

"It does not feel like 'flu."

"You could ring your insurance company for a check-up. In the past people waited until something surfaced. But if it is the case that you want to find out what it is that might surface at some future point . . ."

"It has been going on five nights."

"Drink plenty fluids. Nice to hear from you."

He rings off, which I think offensive. I phone the insurance company. A breezy lady can fit me in next week. "If it is urgent, see a GP."

JUNE

I was brought up in Scotland. We lived ten miles from a village, but a doctor would have visited by this time. Is the

South of England too overpopulated? Is there a different tradition in the North?

A Scots vet, I am certain, would not ignore an animal this long.

It drifts into my mind that Shostakovich, the composer, wrote about bad manners. Rachel finds his *Memoirs*:

> Now I can't abide rudeness . . . Rudeness and cruelty are the qualities I hate most. Rudeness and cruelty are always connected I feel.
>
> (*Testimony*, p. 16)

The wonder here, it seems to me, is the context. Could anyone who lived under Stalin—"Looking back, I see nothing but ruins, only mountains of corpses" (*Testimony*, p. 1)—care about good manners? They must have been an unheard-of luxury. Or were they the real test in that hell? Shostakovich went on:

> As you know, Lenin in his "political will" said that Stalin had only one fault: "rudeness." And that everything else was in good shape . . . And we know how it all ended. No, don't expect anything good from a rude man. And it doesn't matter in what field the boor is.
>
> (*Testimony*, p. 16)

Don't expect anything good from a rude man: it kills the paracetamol doctor for me.

How do I find another doctor? The only doctor Rachel likes is a retired consultant who once treated her for gout. "We know no more about gout than Galen did," he told her—and Galen lived in the ancient Roman Empire. Rachel always warms to experts who confess ignorance. If she gets a chance she cross-examines them until they do. Even if she gets half a chance.

As it happens I met a doctor before I went to Russia, and I liked her. A privilege of my life is that Cameron Mackintosh, the theatre producer, chose me to look after his visiting Professors of Theatre at Oxford. This year it is Peter Shaffer, author of *Equus* and *Amadeus*. He brought his doctor to a lecture and chatted about her: "She has a debby love of fun but can also fix you with 'See that specialist, I've arranged it in one hour's time'—and you know it is life or death."

But there was no trace of grimness when I met Dr. Christian Carritt. In her sixties, beautiful and unelaborately stylish, she had a buoyancy that came from the heart, although you noticed that she did not waste a word.

Still, Dr. Carritt lives in London, which is fifty miles from Oxford. I can scarcely get out of bed.

More nights swimming.

"Dr. Carritt may know of a doctor in Oxford," says Rachel. "We have to do something. You are much too patient."

I phone Dr. Carritt.

"Two weeks sweating? Sounds ghastly. Can someone drive you up to London? Tomorrow. Come to tea. I would like to see you again."

We have tea not in Dr. Carritt's surgery but her sitting room. Prolonged night sweating (I later found out) is a classic symptom of cancer and leukaemias.

"I'd better take some blood."

She does it almost skittishly as we chat about her garden, the theatre, Oxford and Peter Shaffer.

"I'll have this analysed and ring you."

Dr. Carritt phones next day.

"Michael, you are wonderful."

"Wonderful?"

"I cannot understand how you have led a normal life being so anaemic."

"I have been in bed for two weeks."

"No, long before that. Did you have giddy spells?"

In fact, yes. But I put them out of mind: friends, pupils and strangers have been clutched as I steadied myself or fell over. But the giddiness was only for a minute or so. I put it down to not eating. Or tiredness. Or humid weather.

"I have arranged a specialist for you at 9 a.m. tomorrow."

This is said as lightly as offering a sandwich.

"But if it is only anaemia . . ."

"No, you must go."

Not a tone to argue with.

"What shall I tell my doctor?" I ask.

"The last thing people should have to worry about are their doctors. I rang and told him that we met in London, you were not well, and I thought I had better look into it. Now let me know about the specialist. I had to shop around to get one less than a couple of hours from Oxford. Please ring and tell me if they are any good."

This is skill. If you are told to see a specialist next morning, let alone having a specialist searched for, things are bad. But the idea that you, the patient, can help decide the merits of the specialist . . . it distracts from fear and makes the consultation bearable.

"Darling, forgive me if I do not come," says Rachel. "I will only make things worse by being anxious."

The specialist is a senior lady and almost cheerful. A sample is to come from my bone marrow.

"At the end it will hurt like a sting."

It does. I am sent for X-rays.

"They will cost more than I do, I'm afraid. Shall we meet in a week?"

"Not before?"

"I suppose the results can be back tomorrow afternoon."

She smiles indulgently. "The day after at 11 a.m.?"

I go back to the hospital.

The consultant settles behind her desk.

"You have come alone?"

"Yes."

"Do you live alone?"

"No. Why?"

"So there is someone to make a good cup of tea?"

I do not drink tea.

"But are you happy at home?"

"Yes."

She looks doubtful, so I explain that during University term I have lived for twenty years with Rachel.

"Are you very wealthy?"

"No. Poor."

"But you come to me privately."

"I did not want to wait. And I am insured."

"So you are not wealthy?"

"No."

"I just thought you might be thinking of early retirement."

"No. I love my job."

I ask her to bring matters to a head.

"What you have will shorten your life. I cannot say how much. It starts with just one rogue cell. If I knew why, I would get a Nobel Prize. But there is no cure."

"So what is wrong?"

"You have a type of cancer called myeloma. It is a cancer of the bone marrow. Have you heard of it?"

"No."

"Here is a booklet. Are you going to get home all right?"

"I have a taxi."

"Good. I will write to the University. Will you give my secretary the details? That is, if you agree."

"Yes."

"Good. And I would like you in here next week. To start treatment."

"Treatment?"

"Yes. With luck we should have you back at work in October."

"But this is June . . . and you said there was no cure."

"No cure. But we have treatment."

"From next week until October?"

"Yes, and I can tell you the nurses are wonderful."

Crunch time. Decisions. Except the specialist thinks there is nothing to decide. But I am not for humid summers in the South of England, I need hills and fresh air.

Treatment but no cure? Why treat if you cannot cure? Why such a long treatment? And the nurses . . . nurses are wonderful, but they carry out what specialists say. My life is to depend on the intelligence of this lady. She is not explaining what she plans. Even in outline. Am I to sign myself away on nothing? Is that what she expects?

I hear myself saying, "I spend the summers in Scotland."

A couple of minutes pass.

I get up and thank her for her trouble.

She takes a pad, writes and passes me the page.

"What is this?"

"The names of two doctors in Edinburgh."

"Why?"

"They will know what to do if you become immobilised."

Ace of trumps. Played deadpan.

"You think that is likely?"

"Immobilisation is what happens with your cancer."

I still find myself leaving.

"You can always try a second opinion" is the farewell.

I go back to college, not to Rachel's flat. There are roses in the garden. Irises. And moorhens on the river. With a family of blackdown blobs. Fresh air, not the limbo of hospital.

I meet a colleague who asks if it would be easier if he went to Rachel first. I accept his offer, and sit in the sun.

Was I insufferable to the consultant? She was only doing her job. I know nothing about cancer: do I think I am exempt from getting it?

What about the library?

Each Oxford college includes most disciplines, and we take medical students.

I find a book, Rees, Goodman and Bullimore, *Cancer in Practice* (1993). Myeloma is in the index, and p. 193 reads:

> Multiple myeloma is incurable. The median survival time from clinical confirmation to death is under a year in untreated patients, and two to three years with treatment. Some 15% die within the first three months.

Underneath there are:

SYMPTOMS AND SIGNS

Bone pain, pathological fracture, anaemia, symptoms of hypercalcaemia and renal failure, fever due to infection.

So here is my anaemia and fever. Also bone pain: I slipped a disc in 1989, which went on for months, and I am still sore if I sit for any great length of time.

Life as a scholar gives you reflexes. Where does the word *myeloma* come from? Classical Greek? A dictionary gives me Greek *muelos,* bone marrow. Hence *myeloma,* cancer of the bone marrow. Is it a modern disease? The 1991 *Encyclopaedia Britannica* has a villain *myelitis,* also of the bone marrow: "the most that can be hoped for is the relief of symptoms by careful nursing and attention to the condition of the body and its functions."

Myelitis is not myeloma, but the vista of humiliation is enough.

My colleague comes back from Rachel: she asks to be alone for a couple of hours.

Rachel never talks about her fears, and I sometimes think that perhaps she no longer can. If this seems odd in someone so articulate, its source is a great sorrow: Rachel's sister, her only sibling, developed schizophrenia and was institutionalised. However exhausted by work, Rachel would drive hundreds of miles to visit every week. "I have such delight in life and my sister none," Rachel once grieved to me, "and she knows she has none."

I am twenty years younger than Rachel and, although she would not say it, she relies on me to see her out. Now I have cancer.

One of Rachel's best friends was Rosemary Woolf, a scholar of medieval literature who also loved fun and fast cars. They would go on holiday together, driving for weeks in France and Italy. Rosemary developed cancer and Rachel lived with the agonies of Rosemary's treatments, her subsequent falls, illnesses and death.

I forget about ringing Christian Carritt but she phones me while I am still in college.

"Cancer," I say, "bone marrow, though the specialist did not tell me much."

"Do they ever? When I was a student, we were actually trained to tell the patient as little as possible."

"Really?"

"Yes."

I tell her about the book in the library.

"And?"

"Untreated myeloma patients die in less than a year, treated in two to three years."

"Michael, it is very important that you do not take too much notice of statistics. Think how they are calculated. You count up, but every patient is different. One is diagnosed at sixty-eight, another at forty-eight. One might be in the early stages of cancer, another might be diabetic as well. Or depressive. One patient might live in the country, another beside a chlorine plant. Statistics tell you very little about an individual case."

"Is myeloma a rare cancer?"

"No. One of the twenty most common. How was the specialist?"

I go through the consultation. From start to finish: all the way to *immobilisation is what happens with your cancer.*

Silence from Christian.

A long silence.

"My God, what a bully!" she then says. "Were you shown the X-rays?"

"No."

"But why not? Either they do or do not indicate bone about to collapse. If your bones are about to collapse, it will stop you going to Scotland. But my money is on the X-rays showing no such thing."

"Then it is outrageous."

"Yes."

Immobilisation was the trump card of the specialist. Christian now plays a trump of her own. She will arrange a second opinion, of course, but should I not get off to Scotland for a couple of weeks?

And she leaves it there.

No further comment.

"Goodbye."

Bless Christian: she gives Rachel and me something we can bear to talk about. Scotland is dear to Rachel. She thinks it an excellent idea for me to go and she would like to come too, but she grumbles about the lack of comfort in my cottage.

"Michael darling, you are a perfect guest but a tyrannical host."

(In Scotland I try to get her to smoke outside, or in the spare room.)

"And you know, Michael, I am frightened for the dog."

When our dog was a nervous puppy from the strays' home we had taken her to Scotland. She astonished Rachel by leaping from the car and killing a rabbit.

"Suppose," Rachel asks, "she ran away again, chased sheep and a farmer shot her?"

This is an unlikely scenario, but it gets us chatting. We talk about deer, foxes, weasels and snares. Somehow we drift on to bears. I tell Rachel about a circus I went to in Moscow where you could be photographed with a bear who put its paws on your shoulder.

"Muzzled?" asks Rachel.

"Of course."

"Did the bear look healthy?"

"Mangy."

"I hope, Michael, you took no part in this outrage to the bear. Did you have your photograph taken?"

"No."

The rule book would be thrown at me if I had.

Rachel will not come to Scotland: she wants to stay in Oxford and have time to be alone.

Travel is not easy if you are anaemic. You have to think how to do it. Less time, therefore, to think about a death sentence. Looking back, I see that Dr. Carritt's aim was distraction. As simple as that. But distraction is a medicine in itself, as I came to realise. It was common sense, if you like, but never so valuable as when you are not capable of applying it to yourself.

Christian's point was *get away*. A new place will give you new thoughts. And travelling has a rhythm of its own.

She had found my specialist in twenty-four hours. She could find another as quickly. But she did not want to. Instead I was to go to Scotland, because it was what I usually did. This quietly assumed that life might go on as before. The news of a lethal cancer takes you over. But if you can be put back on old tracks somehow, if you can live again according to your own rhythms at least a little, there is a chance for resistances and energies that you have built up over the years.

A chance.

Not that Christian put any of this into words. She was far too skilful: consciousness would add anxiety, which could undermine what might be achieved by instinct.

2

One of my pupils, Rufus Waddington, drives me north. My house in Scotland is a cottage five hundred feet up in the hills of Roxburghshire. The valley below, Liddesdale, was a favourite of Walter Scott and the whole area is still romantic—wild, thinly populated, a land of shepherds and foresters. The snow is horizontal, but there is always the freshness of mountains. Deer browse in gardens when it is bleak, and you hear snipe miles away on a summer night.

The border with England is a mile or so south. There were fierce battles. Hermitage Castle, a grim ruin, guarded the pass to Edinburgh, and at the foot of my hill a sign invites you to "Bloody Bush."

Life in the mountains is still tough. No one thinks they are immortal, but there is little gloom: the days of a shepherd are busy, the hills raise your spirits, the weather has a Western softness but is madly changeable . . . whatever the reason, a sense of fun is just underneath the dry Border ways.

The next stage of my illness may surprise you.

Phone calls.

If this sounds daft, I warn that it may happen to you.

Rachel rings me twice a day and also cross-examines Rufus. "She thinks you will get hysterical," he tells me. But are invalids hysterical? Not as much as people think. Invalid hysteria is one of those concepts that help the world go round, including hospitals: "Keep the patient calm. Do not tell them much. Try love and a tranquilliser." I was to hear a cancer specialist say the last sentence.

Some phone calls are from friends who I thought liked me, but now show they like me very much.

There are also those who phone and ignore your cancer. "What," rings a senior academic, "is going to happen about the Feast in October?" I say I will look after it as usual, if alive. "Fine. Bye."

It is not that he dislikes me or thinks I am about to be mawkish. His energy goes into his work; there is no surplus for thinking about how to talk to someone in crisis. Not but what an element of the stratosphere creeps into University manners.

There are callers who keep on phoning, and at such length you might think they had cancer too. They do not. Peter Selby, Professor of Cancer at the University of Leeds, detects a "morbid glamour" in reactions to cancer (*Confronting Cancer*, p. 3). It is an interesting phrase that he does not develop.

In my case, the morbid glamour operates like this. The caller expresses sympathy. Then a symptom is picked out. What will be the next stage? Treatment is better than it used to be, of course, but what about . . . buds, blossoms, prime sites, lymph nodes, secondaries?

Do not doze off.

You are audience for your caller, and audiences are there to respond.

"Michael, are you taking this as seriously as I am?"

My caller still rang next day.

When I speak to other cancer patients we compare notes about these mini-Draculas. At first I thought they were a guilty secret of mine. "God, no," says one patient, "they are everywhere. I wind them up." In *Before I Say Goodbye,* an account of her own cancer, Ruth Picardie sends this e-mail to a friend who has AIDS but keeps it secret:

> I don't know how you survive without telling the whole world and his aunt about your status—don't you want sympathy, empathy, chocs? I know there's shit involved too, eg endless fucking phone calls demanding detailed analysis of your emotional and physiological state. Sometimes I feel like putting a message on the answerphone. "Hi. Ruth thinks she has secondary bone cancer. Luckily, she is feeling less weepy today (Sunday). Thank you for calling."
>
> (*Before I Say Goodbye,* p. 12)

July, Week 1

Back to London. Christian has arranged a consultation and she comes with me.

Harley Street.

The doctor might have walked in from playing cricket. He is young for his years, sunny and focused. He gives me a general physical examination: eyes, tongue, chest, reflexes and penis. The X-rays and other results have been sent on by the first specialist. (I asked her for them myself, but was refused.) We sit at his desk for the verdict.

"You have got more to offer the world, Mr. Gearin-Tosh. Face up and have treatment. It will not be a holiday, of course. But you should stay around longer. Start the treatment now."

I ask why.

"Cancer is progressive. With myeloma it eats into the bones."

"Is the treatment a cure?"

"No."

"I do not see the point. Suppose I just die of the disease?"

"I would not advise that."

"Why?"

No reply, but he gives a beautiful smile.

"Are you saying I shall have a very painful death?"

"With the drugs we have now, you will not feel a thing."

"So why not die of the disease?"

"Because you should be with us for longer."

"How much longer?"

"Who knows? Research is going on all the time."

"Research into myeloma?"

"Research into all cancers. We may find a cure."

Is this the Ritz of doctorspeak? The glimmer of hope we all like to hear?

The consultant does not have more to say. His desk has been polished with real beeswax, and there is a perfume. The windows are open but it is peaceful and you can only just hear traffic.

I am not going to get ideas from this man: why not ask about facts?

"The X-rays: do they show danger of bone collapse?"

"No."

He catches my eye. "Not that I can see. Of course, it requires an expert to read them."

"And is there an expert's note?"

"I think not."

"Shall we look?"

"I cannot see one."

"May I have the X-rays?"

"I should send them back to Dr. ——— (the first special-ist)."

"They are my property. I paid for them."

He lifts his eyes to Christian. She gives a merry smile.

"I will indicate to Dr. ——— that you would like them sent on."

"Would you say that two years after treatment is my likely survival time?"

"Someone as young and fit as you, Mr. Gearin-Tosh?" He stands up. "I would like you here longer."

I pay the secretary one hundred pounds and leave with Christian.

The traffic is heavy. We avoid Oxford Street and wind through Marylebone. Christian has to go to other patients and there is no time for coffee—it is generous of her to have come at all.

How does she rate the hospital of the Harley Street con-sultant?

"Pleasant as they go. And well run."

"Expensive?"

"Yes. It is London. But your insurance should cover."

A new thought. I ask Christian if I can be sure of the diagnosis.

"There were cancer cells in your bone marrow accord-ing to the first consultant."

"But this man did not check."

"No. He would have had to send samples to a lab. But your immune system was depressed in the blood sample I took, and my analysis was by a different lab from your first consultant."

"So no mistake?"

"Very unlikely. Do you keep a diary?"

"Yes."

"Promise to write fully. It is easy to forget things that turn out to be important."

A friend has offered me her flat in London, which I can use for the summer while she is away. This is convenient for doctors and it also solves a problem about a visitor. When I went to Moscow I wanted to get away from tourist areas but there were reports of mugging. The Theatre Academy found me a bodyguard, no less than a captain in the Russian Army. He was in plain clothes and came with me everywhere. At the end of my trip, I asked if he would like to visit Britain.

"There is no possibility for me."

The captain doubted if the army would allow him to travel, and, in any case, he could not afford the fare.

I said that I would pay: we could set it against my next visit to Russia, if he was prepared to look after me again.

When I got back to England and before my cancer was diagnosed, the captain faxed to say that a visa was possible. Could he come 16–29 July?

"The possibility of travel is the happiest day of my life."

"I cannot face a visitor," says Rachel, "and certainly not a Russian soldier."

She has a prejudice against Russians. "Always a disaster the Slav soul" is her usual pronouncement.

"Why are you letting him come? Two weeks. What on earth can you talk about? You say he slept in plays and ballets. For God's sake, be realistic. Cancel him. Go back to Scotland and rest."

On the last point, Rachel is correct: I would rather be in

Scotland. I phone Moscow. I tell the captain that I have developed a disease of the blood: when he comes, he will have to look after himself.

"Nyet. I look after you."

"London can be humid in July, perhaps you would prefer to visit Scotland?"

"Be in dacha?"

"Yes."

"I am comfortable with twelve hours in dacha and twelve days in London."

I drop any idea of Scotland.

Rachel is opening my mail and the University has sent a letter that they received from my first consultant (*Here are the names of two doctors in Edinburgh in case you become immobilised*):

MICHAEL GEARIN-TOSH

This gentleman, who is a patient of mine, is suffering from multiple myeloma, which will require regular treatment for the rest of his life.

"I thought this consultant said you would be back at work in October," says Rachel.

"She did."

"So she left out the fact that you would be back in hospital again soon after."

Regular treatment for the rest of his life chills us both.

"Did the consultant in Harley Street say you would be permanently in and out of hospital?"

"No."

"God, it is so typical. When I think what Rosemary went through. And others. None were told what would happen.

They had ghastly treatments. Then more ghastly treatments. And in the end? The hospital turns round: 'Nothing more we can do for you. Go home and die.'"

John Diamond, in his heroic account of cancer, *C: Because Cowards Get Cancer Too . . .* , identifies "the principle of gradual disclosure" and maintains that "almost all doctors practise it" (p. 63).

Let the patient find out bit by bit how bad things are.

Rachel also opens a letter from the senior Professor of English Literature, John Carey:

July 6 '94

My dear Michael,

Rachel phoned me last night to tell me what the doctors had said. If there's anything of any kind I can do to help—teaching, etc.—I hope you will let me know at once. We must meet when you are back in Oxford. Do give me a ring so that I can fix a date for lunch or dinner.

With love and best wishes,

Ever,
John.

This is a world apart from the consultant making me think of early retirement.

Two friends visit. I directed them in plays at the Oxford School of Drama and both are now distinguished: Catherine MacCormack, a wonderful actress (Mel Gibson's wife in *Braveheart*), and Mark Miln, a producer.

They know of someone who has just been treated for my cancer, myeloma. The diagnosis is a story in itself. London doctors diagnosed kidney trouble and only after months was cancer found. The patient was so unimpressed that he chose to be treated at the University of Arkansas Cancer Research Center. He made a recording of his initial consultation with its eminent specialist, Dr. Bart Barlogie. If I want, I can have a transcript of the recording.

Yes, please.

Mark brings one round next day.

In the transcript, Dr. Barlogie begins with a clear statement:

> *Barlogie:* The bottom line that everybody agrees upon is that what one considers the conventional treatment for multiple myeloma is not very successful. Patients are not cured with this approach.
>
> *Patient:* Ever?
>
> *Barlogie:* Ever.
>
> (Transcript, pp. 6–7)

In effect, this is what my first consultant said: there is no cure, but we have treatment.

What one considers the conventional treatment for cancers: allow me to try to explain what Dr. Barlogie meant. I shall use information that I did not have at the time. *The conventional treatment* includes chemotherapy. Chemotherapy is a procedure by which poison is put in the blood. No poison, however, attacks only cancer cells and leaves the rest alone. If such a poison existed, it would be magic. But no such luck.

So there are problems.

Dr. Peter Dottino, Head of Gynecological Oncology at Mount Sinai Medical Center, New York, told Liz Tilberis, the editor of *Harper's Bazaar*: "The reason we can't cure cancer is that we can't give enough chemicals without killing the patient. The more chemo we give, the worse havoc we wreak" (Liz Tilberis, *No Time to Die,* p. 8). The "havoc" includes the dreaded side effects: vomiting, "aching veins," hair and eyelashes falling out, saliva not produced, nails falling out. Also, in Liz Tilberis's case, "green moss" growing on her tongue (p. 234) and "my neck swelling like a sumo wrestler's, my lips puffing out like a Ubangi warrior's. My mouth became ulcerated and I could not swallow my own saliva. Every day of chemo brought some new horrifying change to my body" (p. 230).

In attacking cancer with chemotherapy, one dose of poison is not enough. In the words of another authority, Professor Geoffrey R. Weiss of the University of Texas at San Antonio: "It has been well documented experimentally and clinically that anti cancer agents do not destroy all cancer cells following each dose" (*Clinical Oncology,* p. 98). So more doses are given, usually at intervals of two to three weeks. As these doses continue, however, cancer cells may "acquire resistance": "There is a very narrow margin between doses that produce significant toxicity and those that achieve important cancer-killing results. (p. 97). *Significant toxicity* does not mean death, but it comes too close for comfort.

Back to the transcript of the consultation with Dr. Barlogie:

> *Barlogie:* . . . the conventional treatment . . . Patients are not cured with this approach.
>
> *Patient:* Ever?
>
> *Barlogie:* Ever.

Barlogie goes on to consider what doctors are able to do if they go beyond the *conventional treatment.* Bone marrow is the power house of the blood. It is possible to remove some bone marrow before chemotherapy, and the bone marrow can be put back afterwards. Such bone marrow will be undamaged by the chemotherapy poisons, and it can be an aid to recovery. In the words of Dr. Dottino:

> Bone marrow transplant allows us to give an essentially lethal treatment . . . We take out some of your own marrow, freeze it in liquid nitrogen, and when you're sicker than shit, we give it back. We haul you to the brink, push you a bit over, and then pull you back.
>
> *(No Time to Die,* p. 221)

This procedure also allows the doctor to use more poison. Dr. Barlogie describes the process in less feisty language than Dr. Dottino:

> The whole concept behind bone marrow transplantation is to allow the administration of much greater dose intensity in order to kill more cancer cells and to thereby decrcase the tumor burden down to the level where perhaps the immune system can cope with it.
>
> (Transcript, p. 11)

In the transcript, Barlogie says that he is himself "perhaps a little more adventurous in terms of treating than some" (p. 10).

There are doctors who delay putting back the marrow, perhaps for months. They use it if things do not go well, "when your disease can no longer be controlled" (p. 18). But Barlogie puts the marrow back immediately after chemotherapy; "I think one has the best shot up front" (p. 19). And he puts the marrow back in *two* stages, not all at once:

Knowing that myeloma is rather resistant, the treatment one gives with one transplant is not *that* much more effective . . . So we decided OK we will just do two transplants . . . and we have criteria where, if we don't achieve what we want to accomplish after one transplant, we modify the treatment going along with the second transplant, to include total body radiation.

(Transcript, pp. 13–14)

In using two transplants, Barlogie is unique:

Patient: You're the only person doing that?
Barlogie: I think so.

(Transcript, p. 35)

I absorb enough of the Barlogie transcript to be able to talk to Dr. Carritt, and we meet for lunch at a café near her house in South Kensington.

"When was the consultation with Dr. Barlogie?" she asks.

"Two years ago."

"They are new these cancer treatments."

"Is that a vote against them?"

"Dr. Barlogie's patients will be at the front of experiment, but are there long-term side effects from the treatment? There usually are."

"I suppose so."

"It is always a factor to take into account. How is Rachel Trickett taking things?"

"So, so."

"How much older than you is she?"

"Twenty years."

"And anxious?"

"Yes."

"You may have to support her more than she you."

Christian raises a problem that haunts Rachel and me—as it does, I now know, other cancer patients. John Diamond wrote that, "Nobody receives a diagnosis of even the least invasive cancer with anything but fear and dread" and, as a recent textbook observes, "Patients dealing with a diagnosis of myeloma are confronted with a terrifying reality" (Malpas, Bergsagel, Kyle and Anderson, *Myeloma: Biology and Management,* p. 493).

Ideally, those who love each other should be able to explore fear together. But can it ever be easy? How often is it possible?

One of the most poignant moments in *Before I Say Goodbye* is when Matt Seaton, the partner of Ruth Picardie, writes:

> I often felt that, as Ruth was dying, our relationship was by degrees dying with her . . . I just wish—how I wish—I could have somehow got round it: loved Ruth or made her feel loved, in the old way, to the very end. But cancer changed everything: it put us on different tracks, stretching our grasp of one another to the limit and eventually forcing us apart. In the end, I could not reach her, and it felt like a failure in me. And then she was gone.
>
> (pp. 103–4)

You might think that a cancer patient or their loved ones could turn to a doctor for help over fear. But the cancer doctor is in an impossible position. It is a maxim of medicine that "the therapeutic benefits of hope cannot be overstated." So, as part of his or her professional skill, a doctor must try to give hope.

How, then, can the doctor discuss terror?

Yet if the doctor pretends there is no place for fear because all is well, he or she may not be a good liar: patients pick up body language, the overpractised smile, the false tone. Or does the doctor evade the subject of hope? A patient may sense this too.

3

Christian wants to know if a UK hospital has taken up the Barlogie procedure of double marrow transplants. Her first enquiries are not promising. Also, my insurance policy does not cover treatment abroad.

I find out that the cost is $150,000–200,000, "assuming no complications." Too expensive.

So a "cure" exists, but it is only for the rich. I should have worked in the City, not become an academic. Depression.

Despair.

Black days.

I join *Exit.*

The phone rings. It is the richest man I know, and one of the most remarkable. Aru (his full title is Tan Sri Datuk Seri Arumugam) is a self-made Malaysian entrepreneur whom I had met some years before. He is brilliant, creative, always fun and a shrewd observer of the world. I also like his wife, Suguna, and their family very much.

Aru is calling to say hello. I tell him of my cancer. He wants details. I go through the Barlogie story. Without hesitation Aru says, "Go to Barlogie, Michael. I will pay. And travel first-class: tell the clinic to contact me."

It is a fantastic offer.

I talk to Catherine MacCormack and Mark Miln, who gave me the Barlogie transcript. They get in touch with Dr. Barlogie's patient, who in turn phones Dr. Barlogie.

Dr. Barlogie can see me at once: his message is that I should not delay.

Days pass.

I stay in London, walk in Hyde Park and sleep a great deal.

Rachel phones and urges me to action. Aru goes abroad on business, but his PA rings from Kuala Lumpur. She is courteously puzzled. The first consultant said, "Treat now," the second consultant said the same, Barlogie is telling me not to delay, the cancer can only get worse. Should she book a flight to Arkansas?

But I never like to hurry decisions.

My heroes from history include Queen Elizabeth I, who once wrote: "Methinks that I am more beholden to the hinder part of my head than well dare trust the forwards side of the same" (to Burghley, 11 April 1572).

A recent historian calls this a "quaint explanation" of a "near pathological tendency to procrastinate" (Anne Somerset, *Elizabeth I,* p. 280). And so perhaps it is. We procrastinators, however, value the "hinder part" of our heads. It mulls things over at its own pace. You never know what will come out. And when something does, we act on it—often to our own surprise. We are unpredictable, not least to ourselves, and we are the despair of logicians.

Does "the hinder part" of the head also cope with fear? Looking back, I can pick out two tactics, although I gave the matter no thought at the time.

Thoughts floated about in my mind, but if a consultant or friend or anyone else told me to "face up" I switched off. These floating thoughts were more questions than ideas. Why did both the first consultant and Harley Street have this manner of bland non-engagement? Why did the first consultant write to the University in different terms from those she used to me when she indicated the need of regular treatment for the rest of my life? Why was Christian Carritt not pressing me to go to Arkansas?

Also, a phrase of Barlogie's in the transcript stayed with me: *Decrease the tumour burden down to a level where perhaps the immune system can cope with it.* I pick up a *perhaps,* and respect it. Was Barlogie pointing, in his quiet way, to a major question: in what shape is an immune system likely to be after the poisons of chemotherapy?

The second of my tactics in coping with fear is obstinacy. I am not going to Arkansas because I said I would be in London for the visit of the Russian captain.

This is obstinate because the captain is not a particular friend. I invited him to Britain more or less out of good manners. He surprised me with his phrase "the possibility of travel is the happiest day of my life." But, of course, I could postpone his visit.

Václav Havel, the playwright and wonderful dissident who became President of the Czech Republic, wrote letters to his wife from prison. One letter contains this uncharacteristic paragraph:

> Sometimes I have the strangest feeling that I don't really want to leave this place. At least not now. Here you enter a state somewhat akin to hibernation . . . sink into a kind of sweet mental lethargy and the prospect of going back into

the evil world, with its constant demands that you be decisive, becomes somewhat terrifying.

(*Letters to Olga,* p. 29.)

Going to Arkansas would be decisive, London is hibernation and "sweet mental lethargy."

One of my oldest friends rings.

"Sorry about the news, Michael. You okay?"

"Fine."

"What is the plan?"

I have worked with David Ambrose, the novelist and
scriptwriter, so I am tuned to the tones and pace of his
voice. Something is up.

I tell him about the two consultants and Barlogie.

"Have you started anything?"

"Nothing."

"No chemotherapy?"

"No."

"Or radiation?"

"No."

"And you are in pain?"

"No. Just exhausted."

"Anaemia?"

I am surprised that David knows about cancer. He
explains that he has a friend in New York who "happens to
be a cancer authority; in fact, a grand old man of cancer. Former Professor of the Sloan-Kettering Hospital, medal from
the American Cancer Association and so on. Professor Ernst
Wynder. Now works on cancer statistics."

"And?"

"I went through your case with him. 'I tell you one thing,

boy,' he said. 'If your friend touches chemotherapy, he's a goner.' "

Bombshell.

I go back to the Barlogie transcript and I read with ferocity. I must pin down every word.

It is a wonderful idea to record a consultation. Everyone should. How can you listen, really listen, as you sit in a strange room and dice over your own life with a doctor you have not met before?

I see that Barlogie uses words with care:

Barlogie: The first step of any cancer treatment is to achieve what we do refer to as a complete remission.

There is a linguistic signal here: *what we do refer to as* indicates that there is a medical meaning that is different from normal use. I go to a library near the flat. The basic meaning of *remission* is spiritual: it means forgiveness of sin or absolution. But there is also a medical meaning, first recorded in 1685: "A Continual Fever has its times of Remission and Exacerbation, but none of Intermission." The fever lowers, *remission.* It gets worse, *exacerbation.* But no *intermission.* It does not go away. The point is that the disease is not cured: it is a "continual" fever.

The spiritual and medical meanings of *remission* are, in a sense, opposite to each other. Spiritual forgiveness is total: you are cured. But in medical remission you are not cured: the disease is static.

It seems to me that adding *complete* to *remission* increases the problem of misunderstanding. *Complete* suggests the end of struggle and pain, a cure. The reality of remission, however, is aptly put by an American patient in a book that I read later: "remission, that horrible word that denotes it's going to come back" (C. Hirshberg and M. I. Barasch, *Remarkable Recovery,* p. 82).

Doctors might note with regard to these medical words, what Helen Rollason, the sports presenter, wrote about the cancer that was to kill her in 1999:

> Initially my ignorance about cancer was almost boundless. I did not even know what an oncologist was until the day one came to see me. If the question had been thrown at me in a quiz, I would probably have guessed at something to do with pigs.
>
> (*Life's Too Short,* pp. 34–5)

If a BBC professional is unfamiliar with these terms, what hope is there for the general public?

Back to Barlogie. The intellectual kernel of the transcript is the following passage:

> *Barlogie:* Myeloma cancer cells are already resistant. Otherwise one could achieve a complete remission and cure with very simple chemotherapy. Even with transplantation [of bone marrow] when used up front, one does not achieve an 80 per cent complete remission rate. One achieves maybe a 50 per cent complete remission rate.
>
> So half the patients do not go into complete remission and those are clearly the patients who will not be cured.
>
> Out of the 50 per cent who achieve a complete

remission, not all of those have long-term disease control either.

So from my point . . . philosophically, biologically, and all I know about cancer, if this approach of intensive therapy [two bone marrow transplants] is going to work and is actually to generate some long term survivors, then it ought to be used up front and everything ought to be put together to have this chance.

Study these words and hope gets less with every phrase. Fifty per cent get into remission? Not quite. Barlogie said *maybe* fifty per cent. So a bit more than half will not go into remission. These, as Barlogie remarks, *clearly . . . will not be cured.* This means that they will die. *Clearly* is quiet but final.

Am I too sensitive to words, too literary? Do I find death where it is not? I test myself against other pages.

Barlogie: The secret in terms of long-term disease control is not to have a recurrence. Not to have a recurrence. That is the principal law with all cancer. Once the recurrence occurs, the chance to get a cure is minimal. It is going to be shorter and shorter unfortunately.

Recurrence. Not getting into complete remission was, surely, a recurrence. So for more than fifty per cent, who do not get in to complete remission, *unfortunately* is the key word. Ticket on the *Titanic*. Steerage.

Maybe fifty per cent of patients achieve complete remission. But not all will stay that way. Can Barlogie put a figure on it? Does the patient have a forty per cent chance? Thirty per cent? Twenty per cent? What is it, if you listen hard?

Barlogie's words are "*if* this approach . . . is *actually* to generate *some* long-term survivors." Here is a careful man weighing what he says. He will not give a figure. Notice, too, that the word *cure* goes out of his vocabulary as he goes on. At first he talks of "a complete remission and cure." But that was to make an abstract point about what could *not* be done: "*Otherwise* [my italics] one could achieve a complete remission and cure with very simple chemotherapy." As Barlogie deals with reality, *cure* is replaced by "long-term disease control" and "long-term survivors." This is a difference of emphasis. "Out of the 50 per cent who achieve a complete remission, not all of those have *long-term disease control* either . . . if this approach of intensive therapy [two transplants] is going to work and is actually to generate *some long-term survivors.*"

And Barlogie's conclusion is that "everything ought to be put together to have this chance."

Not cure.

Chance.

What does this say about my own consultants? Unlike Barlogie, they were not prepared to take the trouble to sift through these possibilities with me. Result? Bullying (*Immobilisation is what happens with your cancer*) and suave generalisations (*Research is going on into all cancers: we may find a cure*). Easy ways out.

A euphemism of Barlogie's stays with me:

Barlogie: The bottom line that everybody agrees upon is that what one considers the conventional treatment for multiple myeloma is not very successful. Patients are not cured with this approach.

Not very successful: a gentle choice of words, but can failure be more total?

Yet it must be easy for a man of Barlogie's distinction to move to a branch of medicine where cures exist and life is sunny. Not Dr. Barlogie: he is gritting it out.

He is a hero.

I think of a poem by Andrew Marvell, *Upon the Death of the Lord Hastings* (1649). The most famous doctor of the early seventeenth century in France and England was Sir Theodore de Mayerne. He was Court Physician to King Henri IV, and then came to England as doctor to James I and Charles I. There is a wonderful portrait of him by Rubens.

Mayerne's daughter was engaged to Lord Hastings, who was the heir of an aristocratic family. On the very eve of the wedding, Lord Hastings died of smallpox. Marvell pictured the doctor trying to save Hastings's life:

> *But what could he, good man, although he bruis'd*
> *All herbs, and them a thousand ways infus'd?*
> *All he had tried, but all in vain, he saw,*
> *And wept as we, without redress or law.*
> *For man (alas) is but the Heavens' sport;*
> *And art indeed is long, but life is short.*

I spend a couple of days with Rachel before the visit of the Russian captain. She snaps at me, which is a good sign, and means that she has calmed down. This might seem strange to someone who did not know her, but creative irritation is Rachel's usual approach to problems, and, indeed, to much of life.

Her snapping starts when I mention Marvell's poem about Lord Hastings: "For man (alas) is but the Heavens' sport."

"What can you mean, Michael? Man is the sport of doctors, not of God."

She pours a whisky.

"You will remember how Shaw put it."

Rachel knows I do not care for Shaw, of whom she has an encyclopaedic knowledge.

"You know, darling, in the passage about Napoleon."

I also loathe Napoleon, whom Rachel insists on regarding as sexy.

Flushed at the prospect of a fight, Rachel finds a copy of Shaw's play *The Doctor's Dilemma.* It has a long preface that she starts to read: "The medical profession is a murderous absurdity . . . which practises the most revolting cruelties in the pursuit of knowledge."

"My God, that puts it," she says. "I often ask candidates for Oxford: why have doctors always been satirised? And, Michael, why have they?"

"But Rachel, I think some doctors are wonderful."

"The clever candidates always get it right: doctors are hated because they play at being God."

She reads on:

Napoleon had no illusions about doctors; but he had to die under their treatment . . . In this predicament most people fall back on the old rule that if you cannot have what you believe in, you must believe in what you have . . .

Suppose, for example, a royal personage gets something wrong with his throat, or has a pain in his inside. If a doctor effects some cure with a wet compress or a peppermint lozenge nobody takes the least notice of him. But if he operates on the throat and kills the patient, or extirpates an internal organ and keeps the whole nation palpitating for days whilst the patient hovers in pain and fever between life and death, his fortune is made . . .

When Florence Nightingale said bluntly that if you overcrowded your soldiers in dirty quarters there would be an outbreak of smallpox among them, she was snubbed as an ignorant female who did not know that smallpox [did Shaw mean typhoid?] can be produced only by the importation of its specific microbe.

"Shaw is so much more intelligent than Chekhov," says Rachel, "and better informed."

She knows I love Chekhov and that I also value the fact that Chekhov was a doctor, and a practising doctor, as well as a writer.

Rachel is letting off steam, and I now find why. She is opening my mail and she has come across a letter from a pupil of twenty years ago.

Carmen Wheatley has heard I am ill. She rang a couple of days ago, and then wrote as follows:

12 July

Dear Michael,

If you have to die, I am sure no one will do it better. And if you have decided you want to die, that is fine. But I have a profound objection to physicians who deliver death sentences.

How can your consultant know what is going to kill you? There are so many variables in the course of a disease. Even with something as dire as Aids, there are cures—even if unexplained.

I am convinced that, the will of God apart, what happens next is much more in your hands than you might suppose. I do not know what your thoughts are on the subject. But the power of mind over matter is almost magical, if you have once experienced it.

Dennis is not a bad example [Dennis Horgan, my senior colleague]. He has been dying twenty years, when most normal people would have fallen at the first hurdle. And we cannot have him outliving you . . . You have always been so strong and vital, I am sure you have great resources.

Forgive me, Michael, if I am adopting a hectoring, evangelising tone. It may be inappropriate, and I can almost see you wincing. But I have a suspicion that you give too much weight to your consultants' words, are already planning your funeral party, and may be leaving any decisions till after the summer when you could well have lost critical ground.

If I were you I would want to collect the maximum amount of information on your condition now and evaluate all possible avenues of treatment now. Get hold of the medical text books, papers etc.

I hope that you will get further opinions sooner rather than later, and preferably in the next week or two. I have written to a friend who is a doctor to see who he would recommend.

But finally remember that doctors can be very fallible. To give you a personal example, eight years ago Charlie [Carmen's partner, Dr. Charles Lane, a biochemist] was diagnosed as having a brain tumour, by a very reputable Harley Street man. He was given the news in a waiting room full of patients. It took us several months of alternative opinion seeking, and two trips to the States for tests and scans, to establish that it was a false diagnosis. You can imagine what life was like till then.

If Charlie had gone along unquestioningly with that consultant, he would have been subjected to some dangerous and potentially life-threatening tests and treatment.

Charlie is trying to track down some information on the latest treatments for myeloma in America from his oncologist con-

*tacts there. I will forward anything as soon as I have it. I am
also going to ring one of my oldest friends, an anaesthetist with
a special interest in pain relief, to see if he has anything to offer.
But let us hope you will not need that.*

*If there is anything else that I can do, just call. I do have a
beautiful upstairs room with a balcony and view over Wychwood
Forest. It is quite separate from the main house, and if you
need a rest, you are welcome here anytime, for as long as you like,
with or without a friend. You would be well cared for!*

> *Much love,*
> *and take very good care,*
> *Carmen*

It is a wonderful letter.

"Outrageous," says Rachel. "The girl is not a doctor. You
always think too highly of your pupils and believe they are
more gifted than they are. She may be very beautiful . . ."

"Carmen is very clever."

"What can you mean? Cleverness only means anything if
you are competent. She has no medical training. Here she is
putting you in touch with more doctors. You have too many
of the damned things already. Does she expect you to spend
'several months of alternative opinion seeking'? You will be
dead. As for this other woman you value so much . . ."

She means Christian Carritt.

"Has she told you to get on with anything?"

"No."

"What do these society doctors do? Sit on the fence. You
might as well meet her for a cocktail. 'See how things go.
Will you be at Ascot?' And you pay a hundred pounds."

"In fact Christian has not asked me for a penny."

"So she likes you. What the hell does that have to do
with cancer?"

•   •   •

In Rachel's moods there is excitement as well as assertion: she is like a Rossini overture with crescendo and vibrato, and what she needs is someone who does not dive for cover.

I let the storm run its course.

"At least, darling," she now laughs, "your life does not change."

"I have cancer. My stomach is awful. I cannot take tea or coffee."

"Could not happen to a better person. You always had fads: you can let them take you over. What I said was that your life does not change. Three bossy women, and you take the advice of none of them."

"But Carmen has only sent a letter."

"That is not a letter: it is a programme. She will be at you every day."

Rachel triumphs when another letter comes from Carmen next morning:

13 July

Michael,

  A good man for pain treatment is Dr. —— who works at the pain relief clinic at the Churchill Hospital. Obviously your doctor should make the referral.

Love,
Carmen.

"It is going to be me, Carmen and Christian Carritt," says Rachel.

"If any of you has the answer to cancer . . ."

"Darling, a reason why I love you is that you listen to advice, but you have a talent for not taking it."

"Stop it. I think all four of us are rebels."

"What can you mean? Me a rebel? I ran a college of the University of Oxford."

I first met Carmen because she was rebelling against Rachel and Rachel's college. Everyone was out of bounds. Carmen applied to Oxford to study languages. She sailed through the interviews (her mother is Spanish and Carmen is bilingual). She was offered a scholarship in languages but then said that she wished to study English Literature.

Rachel put her foot down and insisted that Carmen at once sit the full examinations in English Literature. Two three-hour papers. To be written that day.

Carmen had heard that you were offered sherry by Oxford professors.

None so far.

She asked for a bottle while she wrote, and drank another in the second exam.

I have never found out what happened next—nor how much all this was a myth which grew—but there was no place for Carmen at Rachel's college.

We accepted Carmen at my college, St Catherine's and, three years later, she took a first-class degree. She then wrote a thesis on Donne and Spanish Literature, supervised by John Carey—hence Carmen is *Dr.* Wheatley. But she did not follow an academic career. She left Oxford and became the consort of Dr. Charles Lane, a molecular biologist.

Another letter from Carmen:

Dear Michael,

Keep your spirits up. I will not let you die of ignorance.

Some books and articles will come under separate cover. If you master the outlines of your condition, it will help when you speak to consultants.

For general information, note the chapter on "Plasma Cell Tumours" in Cancer Medicine *2 (1993), pp. 2075–6.*

Complications of Cancer Management *may be in the gloom and doom camp but could be useful if you have a bone marrow transplant: pp. 41–62.*

Ideally, if I were you, I would locate a medical student, with a first, and commission them/him/her to do a few days' research for you, summing up your options and pitfalls, and providing you with photo-copies of relevant literature, on all therapies available—phototherapy and hyperthermic therapy included, as well as US developments.

I'd be happy to sponsor this for you, if it is of any use to you.

Let me know if I can help but I am just an amateur hypochondriac.

> *Much love,*
> *Carmen.*

"It is role reversal," says Rachel, "she is treating you like a student."

"What a wonderful idea."

"Do not be absurd. But, if you want to be her pupil, shall I unpack *Complications of Cancer Management*?"

Rachel then seizes *Complications of Cancer Management* and starts to read it herself.

I am left with a paperback by Dr. Jan de Vries, *Cancer and Leukaemia*.

In one of his chapters, Dr. de Vries quotes the Bible: "King Solomon also wrote: 'Being cheerful keeps you healthy. It is slow death to be gloomy all the time' (Proverbs 17:22)."

"Cannot leave the Bible alone," interrupts Rachel: she is

only pretending to read *Complications of Cancer Management* in order to keep it from me for as long as she can.

She fetches the traditional King James translation of the Bible. There the verse is: "A merry heart doeth good like a medicine: but a broken spirit drieth the bones."

"You see," Rachel declares. "The King James Version puts medicine in a sane context. We can all identify with *a merry heart*. But de Vries's *slow death to be gloomy all the time* . . . the dowdiness of modern truism."

The traditional Bible's phrase *drieth the bones* interests me. In myeloma, the cancer eats into the bones. If you do not die in any other way, your skeleton collapses.

The idea of drying the bones is absent from the translation de Vries uses, but later in his book he writes that "the Chinese believe that the centre of your bones is responsible for the well being of the body as a whole" (pp. 149–50).

New idea to me. And de Vries goes on to describe a Chinese bone breathing exercise.

Could it be on target for bone marrow cancer? Worth a try. I leave Rachel and go to another room. The exercise is very elaborate. Truly Chinese? I lie on my back, feet apart, arms by my side, palms up. Calm breathing for a few minutes.

I am then to imagine breath coming in through the toes of my left foot and up the bones of the left leg to the hip. Then breathe out from the hip along the same route. In and up, out and down, seven times. Same procedure with the right leg. In and up, out and down, seven times. Back again to the left. Breath comes in through the left foot, up to the left hip and now across to the right hip. You breathe out down the right side. The shape of a U. Seven times.

I then breathe in through the fingers of my left hand up to the shoulder. Breathe out from the shoulder down to the fingers. Seven times. Ditto with the right hand. Seven times. U movements again: up from the left hand to the left shoulder and across to the right shoulder, breathe out down the right arm. Seven times. Same procedure in reverse, right hand, right shoulder, across to left and out. Seven times.

The spine. Breathing in, I go to the top; breathing out, to the base. Seven times. Same with the skull—this feels the most odd. Seven times. The final breathing starts with both feet and goes through all the bones to the top of the skull. All the time, breathing in. Then down again in a giant breath out. Up. Down. Seven times.

At the end I am deliciously warm and so airy I can float.

The book says that cancer patients "should do such an exercise three times a day."

It is all only part one of the exercise: there is a further section of mental visualisation.

Rachel bursts in.

"You tell me that you breathe through your toes?"

Best to leave the visualisation section for now.

4

I meet the Russian captain at Heathrow and we go to a fish restaurant. He examines the menu as if it was illegal and growls, "McDonald's." Steak is found and he drinks beer.

Back at the flat, he inspects the fridge. My shopping passes muster.

Next morning, real breakfast: sausage, bacon, herring and vodka.

"Now I smoke."

There is a balcony in the flat, God be thanked. The Captain has brought a tent mat. (Why? Habit? Is it for the street, in case I prove intolerable to live with?) The mat is unrolled. He has brought enough cigarettes for the fortnight. On each packet a single woodbine fumigates Russia up to the Urals.

An hour later, he leaves with a map of central London:

"Bye-bye, sweetie. Tonight I make you borsch."

I try to stay awake—it is now only 9 a.m.—but I next surface in the afternoon.

The captain comes back in the evening.

"Borsch."

There is military precision. An onion is put in boiling

57

water for twenty minutes. Then out. Timed exactly. Potatoes and cabbage, cut up, are put in for five then grated beetroot and carrot in the proportion four to two, finely cut peppers in the proportion three to the preceding, and as many tomatoes as possible. Boil fifteen minutes. Chopped parsley, spring onions, herbs and a whole plate of garlic—pressed—are added for thirty seconds only. Heat off. The borsch is to sit for an hour.

"In camp there is pig's knuckle."

I explain that my illness has turned me off meat. And salt.

"Name of illness?"

"Myeloma."

"Write please."

I ask how his day had been.

"Nyet. Now English lesson."

This is a surprise. The captain has not mentioned English lessons, but I am happy to oblige, although I say that he speaks English well.

"You are not serious man."

He brings out his Petersburg Military Academy English book. It begins with drawings of where the tongue should be for each sound. They are large anatomical illustrations, with teeth, tongue muscles, etc. I have never seen anything like them. The drawings go on and on, page after page.

"No words?" I ask.

"First, positions."

I think back to the Russian Academy of Theatre Arts: "Our students do not open their mouths until they study the throat and larynx." And when the Maryinsky or Kirov ballet schools hold auditions, the streets are jammed with families from all over Russia. Such training. Such standards. But the methods . . . not the world of Pushkin in 1830 where "we all meandered through our schooling haphazard" (*Eugene Onegin,* Chapter 1, Canto 5).

There are phrases in the captain's book, and short conversations:

> I did not hear the phone because I was listening to folk music on the radio.

and

> I like the rhythm of this overture.
> So do I. But the whole sounds like an amateur performance.
> Anyhow, it's drawing to a close.

The captain asks me to check his pronunciation.

> Is sugar rationed as well?
> Yes, and the rations are smaller for adults.
> How much are the adult persons getting?

> I choose the wrong moment to giggle.
> "You laugh at my country?"
> "But rationing stopped many years ago in Europe."
> "Russia is not Europe? Are you comfortable with this idea?"

The captain is off before I wake up. I do a breathing exercise and walk to an organic shop for vegetables. To my surprise I do not take a taxi back, but walk for a good hour.

Aerated bones?

I ask the captain if he would prefer to go to a restaurant some nights.

"Money for doctors. Learn borsch."

This is said without humour. And I do not smile during the English lesson:

Shall I make her a bouquet?
Of course. Cut a dozen dahlias.
Where are the scissors?
In the top drawer of the cupboard.

My old friends Gillie and Patrick Sergeant are in town and their daughter Emma Sergeant, the painter, recommends a healer who has helped her. Carol Bosiger stimulates reflexes on my feet in order to "balance energy flows" through the body. She also tells me to change my diet: 75 per cent vegetables each day and in particular avocados, beans, beetroot, carrots, garlic, lettuce and onions.

No coffee, tea, salt, sugar, sweets, preservatives, tomatoes and white flour. And no alcohol.

I should also take vitamin C and build up to the highest point I can tolerate "without getting the runs." And she recommends an herbal preparation to boost my immune system.

Carol's diet fits Igor's borsch apart from the tomatoes, which I quietly drop from my shopping.

A few days later, the captain returns at lunchtime. He is out of film and wants to take the cards in a phone booth.

"In Moscow nobody will believe."

We go out together. He photos a black cab—"like museum"—and he lies on the pavement to take a "sky-scrapper."

There is a shop with a sale.

"Can I go in?"

"Of course."

"But I will not buy."

"It does not matter."

"In Russia we stand in line and are shown products. I am embarrassed to leave and not buy. It is out of my expectation."

"Just say you are looking around."

"I must remember this words."

I ask if he is lonely as he sightsees each day.

"Do not be sorry. I meet friends. Russians."

"Did you know them before?"

"No. Shoes."

"Shoes?"

"The whole of Russia wears these terrible shoes. All same. Brand *Salamander.* I see one man in Trafalgar Square. 'Hello?' Yes. He is Russian. Maxim. We have a beer."

Another letter comes from Carmen:

20 July

Michael,

The following is the most useful and encouraging information I've found so far. I hope it will help:—Charlie reached Steve P., who is the No. 2 at a bio-tech company with a very high-calibre team of scientists attached. He lost his wife about ten years back, as a result of myeloma. Ironically, she died not of the cancer, but of an opportunistic pneumonia, just after she had responded very successfully to treatment.

In Steve's view there are three centres of excellence for your cancer in the US.

1)   The Dana Farber Cancer Centre in Boston.

2)   The M. D. Andersen Hospital in Texas.

3)   The Mayo Clinic.

What happens is that your own healthy marrow is extracted, treated and stored. In the meantime you are treated by a chemotherapy cocktail and possibly some radiotherapy. Then your bone marrow is reintroduced, and if all goes well, you are as good as new. This is actually what Steve's wife did. It is just bad luck she succumbed to pneumonia, which ten years on, could have been prevented by a prophylactic antibiotic spray, recently available. Perhaps you should get your medical student to find out the exact chemotherapy regime used at Dana Farber, and replicate it here in the UK, under your insurance.

Love

Carmen.

I know about the bone marrow extraction from Barlogie, but I do not like some of the words in Carmen's letter. I guess she is passing them on from Mr. P., and Mr. P. is repeating what came from his wife's doctors. *She died not of the cancer, but of an opportunistic pneumonia, just after she had responded very successfully to treatment.*

Very successfully?

Did tests show that cancer factors were in remission? Perhaps all cancer factors were, and in complete remission. But if you then die of pneumonia ... What does that say?

And what is "opportunistic" pneumonia? Is there a medical meaning as in *complete remission*? I go out to a library and consult the full *Oxford English Dictionary.* There is no special meaning. "Opportunistic" is like "opportunism":

A term first of Italian and then of French politics, which in English use has been extended to characterise any method or course of action by which a party or person adapts him-

self to, and seeks to make profitable use of, the circumstances of the moment.

A party or person adapts himself . . . Or a germ adapts itself.
A micro-organism. A pneumonia. And kills you.

When I am back home, it strikes me that the question to
ask is: can there be opportunism without an opportunity?

All Mrs. P.'s doctors line up in front of me. GP, oncologist,
myeloma expert, marrow transplant surgeon, anaesthetist,
everyone. All are male and in white coats, except for the GP,
who wears a suit, with too youthful a tie. Nobody is to
leave until I finish my post-mortem.

Good afternoon. Why did Mrs. P. die? Gentlemen, we all
know that pneumonia is not an answer because the pneumonia was *opportunistic.* The question is what gave an opportunity to the opportunistic pneumonia.

Cancer?

But you have just given Mrs. P. *very successful treatment* for
cancer. So it was not cancer. Did she have a disease in addition to cancer? Did this additional disease so weaken her that
pneumonia killed her? That would be an opportunity. The
additional disease must have been very serious to have this
effect after your *very successful treatment* for cancer. Tests will
have picked it up.

No.

No?

No.

But that leaves only one possibility. If she did not die of
cancer, if she did not die of an additional disease, she must
have died of your treatment. Yes, your treatment. Your treatment weakened her to such an extent that the pneumonia
got its opportunity. And, as we know, she died *just after* your

very successful treatment. Not years after, not months after, but *just after.*

I do not notice the captain coming back in the middle of this conversation.

"You have mobile phone, Michael?"

"No. I am talking to myself about my cancer."

He goes to the kitchen while I look through some of the books that Carmen has sent. In Geoffrey R. Weiss, *Clinical Oncology,* p. 355, I find: "Immunocompromised patients are subject to a host of bacterial, fungal, viral and other opportunistic infections."

Mrs. P.

To a tee.

Next day, Igor—the captain—insists on coming with me to Carol Bosiger. She is on holiday but sees me at her home in Kent.

I take the letter from my first consultant (*Here are the names of two doctors in Edinburgh*):

Michael Gearin-Tosh

   This gentleman, who is a patient of mine, is suffering from multiple myeloma, which will require regular treatment for the rest of his life.

"Tear it up," says Carol, "these people know nothing."

I ask why, but she will not expand. Nor do I get round to asking what she thought of opportunistic pneumonias.

Igor spends the whole day with me, and the next. But he does not explain his change of routine. It is only as I write, seven years later, that he tells me what happened. When he came to London he asked for the name of my disease. I wrote *myeloma,* which was not in his dictionary. But when I was fantasising over Mrs. P., I said *cancer.*

"I was appalled. For me, cancer means death. From then on, I was always looking at you. I will not see him again, I thought. I tried to say something every day, but I could not find words."

Christian Carritt comes back from holiday and I bring her up to date with Wynder: *If he touches chemotherapy he is a goner.*

"After all the attention that you gave to the Barlogie transcript, Michael, I would explode at the contradiction."

"I did explode, but about something else."

"What?"

I show her Carmen's letter about Mrs. P. and opportunistic pneumonia.

"Surely Mrs. P. died of the cancer treatment?" I say.

"No," Christian replies, "she died of pneumonia."

"Opportunistic pneumonia from the opportunity of the cancer treatment."

Christian thinks I am being obsessive, and changes the subject.

"What about the Russian captain? Do you go to parties?"

"I can just about go for a walk. He makes friends. He sees London. And we have English lessons."

"I bet he has a whale of a time."

"Bit dull."

"Try not to be alone when he goes. I am sure we both like our own company. But it is not good in the stress you are going through."

I go back to the subject of Mrs. P. "Christian, in his transcript Barlogie said—after all the careful calculations, expertise, the double transplant and so on—'The whole concept is to decrease the tumour burden down to where perhaps the immune system can cope with it.' But if that is *the whole concept* and an 'opportunistic pneumonia' can kill you within days . . ."

"Of course. It is cruel."

"The immune system is wrecked by the cancer treatment?"

"It is a balance."

"Sounds like life and death."

"Michael, I want you to have a treatment that you are happy with. Shall I take blood and see how you are doing?"

The Chinese breathing exercise is a combination of stretching and relaxation. Or so it seems. You stretch internally—dare I write, you stretch where other parts cannot reach. And the exercise is a combination. It is not stretching followed by relaxation: the two are astonishingly simultaneous.

I decide this time to try the mental visualisation, which is the second part of the exercise. De Vries's instructions are:

> imagine that you see your cancer cells. See them as they really are: sickly, weak cells, more bone than flesh, whose only power lies in hiding from the immune system, but who cannot really fight back. And now imagine strong, powerful, purposeful white bloodcells. They come right on, like soldiers on the march. They attack the sickly cells.
>
> (*Cancer and Leukaemia,* p. 152)

Like soldiers on the march.

Igor, where are you?

Out sightseeing.

But I can think Russian. I give my cells borsch. Made military: with pigs' knuckles, like it should be. And salt. Rich fleshy stew.

Hang on.

The book says that the killer cells are strong, powerful, purposeful *white* blood cells. White was the uniform of the Czars. A communist Red Army captain will shoot me.

But if you are able to breathe through your toes . . . I order my troops into battledress for snow combat.

In the evening, Igor tells me about his childhood. He grew up on a collective farm in the Stavropol Region, North Caucasus.

"We were both lucky," I say.

I describe the farm in Scotland on which I was brought up, how we would get up before dawn to shoot wild geese, or burn bracken on the winter hills.

"The collective was disgusting," says Igor. "My God, you cannot imagine. Thirty kilometres from anywhere. Road too muddy for use five months. There was no river. Hot wind all summer. How could we breathe? By making a dark room with newspapers over the window . . . All we dreamed of was getting away."

Gunshot. In the flat? What the . . . Igor is on the kitchen floor.

Suicide?

Stop.

It is 6 a.m. I am awake. There is no smell of shot, and there is a smell of breakfast.

How hard do you dare slap a captain in the Russian Army?

I go for it.

Within seconds, a champagne bottle is on Igor's lips.

"Michael, tonight I train you in borsch."

"Why?"

"Do you sleep twenty-four hours? On Sunday I fly Moscow. I train you today. Friday you cook borsch. Saturday I get drunk."

I have lost count of time.

Can I get him a present as a farewell?

"Da."

We go to Selfridges. Igor wants sunglasses.

They are inspected as if they are weapons on which life depends.

"One hundred pounds, sir."

"Nyet."

"Yes, one hundred pounds," says the assistant.

I say that I will pay.

"Nyet. Not serious."

As we walk out, Igor says that he has learned something.

"Decadent madness of fashion?" I ask.

"Nyet. I learn that I have taste."

Benjamin Ross comes to visit while Igor is out. Benjamin was my pupil at Oxford ten years ago. The University teaches English Literature and many other subjects by a system of one-to-one tutorials. Each week a student completes written work and takes it to a tutor. Tutor and student sit together for an hour and examine the work.

Like many graduates of Oxford, I can still remember my tutors. "Answers are not the challenge," Freddy Bateson sighed, "try to ask questions." "Three half points, you idiot, never add up to a point," John Sparrow would say. The tutorial system is daunting—and for both sides: nobody is more ruthless than the student who spots a flaw or a slide in a tutor's arguments. If much can be achieved intellectually, the system, in my experience, is too strenuous for friendship, which, if it occurs, comes later. Often after many years, as between Carmen and me. But there are exceptions.

I was forty-two and Benjamin Ross eighteen when he came to Oxford. Benjamin, however, asked me to a movie in his first weeks. We got into the habit of seeing each other often, and I found that he was one of the people who I most like to talk to.

Even at eighteen, Benjamin was certain that he wished to become a film director. But he had decided to study literature first. He was pleased to see in my room, an autograph that Jean Renoir, the great director, wrote for me:

If a student asked me how he should become a film director, I would tell him to study the great authors, Shakespeare, Milton, Chaucer, Molière, Rabelais, Dante, Virgil, Goethe, Aristophanes and so many others who helped to build a bridge between ourselves and the world.

Jean Renoir
Oxford, 27 of November, 1967

Benjamin took a first-class honours degree in English Literature at Oxford in 1985, and he then went to Columbia Film School. His first film was *The Young Poisoner's Handbook* (1995) with Hugh O'Conor and Tony Sher. Now, as I write, I have come from his second film *RKO 281* with John Malkovich, Harriet Walter, David Suchet and Fiona Shaw.

The stars of the London premiere, however, were Ben's wife Kate and their daughter Alfie.

Back to the events of my cancer, which are some years before Ben's marriage.

On the afternoon in July when I see Ben he has just suffered a tragedy. He is in love with Kate Hill, a different Kate from his future wife, whom he had not yet met. One night as they make love, she has a brain haemorrhage, then dies hours later. The funeral was yesterday.

It is Igor's last night and he goes off to get drunk.

Back at 4 a.m. Upright. He could go on parade. And when we leave for the airport, he is the Russian captain again, unsmiling.

5

"Try not to be alone when the captain goes." Christian gave me wise advice but I ignore it.

I am also shattered by Benjamin's suffering.

My diary is incoherent for the following days, so I write in the past tense.

Alone in the flat in London, I was skimming through one of Carmen's books and I came across an account of medical training:

There was a lecture given by a French Professor and it was followed by a question and answer session.

I remember one of my colleagues asking an unusual question and the Professor responded by asking why she should want to pose that particular one. She then replied that she herself had cancer. Immediately the Professor reacted: "Please do not ever use the word cancer again. When you put it like that, you influence yourself negatively and make your problems worse."

Do not ever use the word cancer again: so you are not allowed to name what is killing you?

The Professor stepped on a landmine in my psyche.

Naming the facts *makes your problem worse*? I had read somewhere that there were Holocaust victims who paid to go in first-class trains to the camps. I imagine the French cancer Professor on the trains and I hear him yelling through a loudspeaker, "Do not think you are on a journey. Do not ever use that word journey again. You influence yourselves negatively, and make your problems worse."

Primo Levi wrote that "everybody has a duty to reflect on the Holocaust," but for my generation the images are in our veins. If you read *Before I Say Goodbye,* you will love Ruth Picardie: she lives in the pages as generous, adventurous, down-to-earth, loving and sane. Yet in her final weeks she wrote: "Am particularly interested in how Holocaust victims contemplated death." She was in London with her husband, her children, love and every medical care. But cancer had taken her mind to terror.

I, too, was in London, but I now saw children's clothes on fences. It is a detail, unforgettable for anyone who knows his great testament, from the night before Primo Levi was sent to Auschwitz:

> And night came, and it was such a night that one knew that human eyes would not witness it and survive. Everyone felt this: not one of the guards, neither Italian nor German, had the courage to come and see what men do when they know they have to die.
>
> All took leave from life in the manner which most suited them. Some praying, some deliberately drunk, others lustfully intoxicated for the last time. But the mothers stayed up to prepare the food for the journey with tender

care, and washed their children and packed the luggage; and at dawn the barbed wire was full of children's washing hung out in the wind to dry.

(*If This Is a Man,* p. 21)

Another image surfaced, probably because the cancer Professor was French. In Losey's film *Mr. Klein* trains hurtle from occupied Paris. Train after train. To the camps.

I doubt if I had thought of the film for twenty years, but now I could not get rid of the noise.

I went through a depression many years before. Foolishly, perhaps, I have never been to a psychiatrist or counsellor. But such an experience stays with you.

I decided that I must act quickly. I had the idea that the trains were drowning out worse noises: I did not want to hear the camps. The only way to stop the noise, I thought, was to listen to real trains.

So I walked to Paddington station.

Quiet at 3 a.m.

I waited for trains to come but I got cold.

I walked to another station.

Charing Cross was also quiet, so I walked in the Strand. Then I saw a wino, and he sparked off memories.

One night in Moscow, I had been bored with a play and left during the interval. As Igor and I took our coats, a lady stood in front of us.

"But everybody loves the second half. Why are you leaving?"

I replied that I would prefer to visit a railway station.

The fact was that I had been thinking for a couple of days that stations were good places to watch people. But my remark was absent-minded, and, of course, it was not the thing to say.

"Inform me what you did not like," the lady asked.

I said that the actors were not concentrating, the lighting cues were slack, the co-ordination of music and action was careless. I tried to answer her question, as idiot academics will.

She heard me out.

"I will see that everyone is in my office after the performance and gives an explanation."

I fled from the theatre, but I thought that the least I could do was go to a railway station. Now Igor was obstructive.

"Nyet railway station. I am ashamed."

"I have embarrassed you?" I replied. "I am sorry."

"Nyet. In railway station you see filthy people. Drunks."

"London stations are as bad."

"I do not believe."

In the end, Igor agreed to take me to the station for Belarus. There was a line of men and women selling things, biscuits, bread, oranges, paper towels—anything to make a little money.

Also there was a drunk. He was upright. Not singing or spitting.

Igor marched over.

The drunk listened to Igor's remarks, which lasted for some minutes.

The drunk moved off, respectfully.

"Did you see?" said Igor. "My God, a disgrace. He had pissed himself."

The trains to Belarus were enormously long, and built to go through temperatures of minus twenty to thirty degrees: people were boarding for Minsk with bags of food, thermoses and blankets.

We passed a stairway in the station.

"Nyet for visitors," said Igor.

But it was a public stairway: could I not go up?

At the top there were seats and hundreds of people.

"Are they waiting for trains?"

"These people come Moscow to buy what is not in towns. No money for hotel, so they spend nights here."

"How long will they stay?"

"What it must take."

I travelled on a train in Russia. The Principal of the Theatre Academy, Sergei Issayev, took me on the famous overnight train to St. Petersburg.

We had dinner before we left, and Issayev brought two friends who were to travel with us so that we would fill a sleeping compartment. There was course after course of zakuski: fish with horseradish, ox cheek in aspic, beetroot caviare, cheeses from the Ukraine, pizzas—Russians claim to have invented them—and vodka so cold there was ice on the bottle. Next morning we were to leave the train on an empty stomach and into bitter fog.

There were dogs on the Petersburg platform. Families brought them like friends. A cocker spaniel, borzois and huge wolfhounds. Solzhenitsyn wrote:

> Nowadays we do not think much of a man's love for an animal; we laugh at people who are attached to cats. But if we stop loving animals, are not we bound to stop loving humans too?

These were the memories that came back as I stood in London near Charing Cross station. Not much logic, but the massive trains stood for resistance. Only against the cold. But resistance.

And the lines of people at the Belarus station . . . "They come from other parts of Moscow," Igor said, "because they are ashamed to be seen selling. They make a few kopecks from a packet of biscuits." So the lines of people stood for struggle, as did those who sat up all night in the cold railway station.

Of course, these images were not in a context of horror, let alone Nazi horror. Nor were they comparable to the unspeakable courage and love of the mothers who washed the children's clothes on that night of terror. But I doubt if I could live with such intensity of terror and also fight cancer. I needed the images to transpose themselves to gentle forms.

The French cancer Professor, however, and the Nazi trains are to haunt me for weeks to come.

I must go to Scotland, but I am still too raw: I cannot face being in a train.

Perhaps I should buy a car.

Why not?

My friend Shawais, a Kurdish refugee, sells me an old Mercedes and offers to drive it to Scotland "to show that it works."

Rachel only buys new cars: "It cost seven hundred and fifty pounds? For God's sake, Michael, join the AA: they have a breakdown service."

"Are you running away?" asks Carmen.

She thinks I will stay in Scotland and put everything off until the University term starts in October. Am I remembering, she asks, the appointment in Oxford she has arranged with Dr. Littlewood, a cancer clinician and researcher?

I say that a month ago she accused me of planning to die.

"So the programme is now picnics?" she replies.

I assure Carmen that I will come back for Dr. Little-wood.

"An old banger, but enormous," says Christian when she sees my car. And it is large next to the Kensington BMWs.

Christian tells me that my blood results are better: the haemoglobin levels are:

17 June	9.4
24 June	10.2
28 July	11.3

The normal male level is 14–18, so I am well below par. But the trend is in the right direction.

Helen Rollason also bought a car:

> just when I was beginning to despair about my cancer, I splashed out more than I have ever spent on anything with less than three bedrooms—a flash new Mercedes Roadster. "What the hell. I have got cancer. I am allowed to do this sort of thing. It is my pension."

Is movement irresistible when you may have to give it up?

August Week 2

We drive 350 miles to Scotland without trouble, although Shawais speeds less than in his own modern car.

Scotland is hot. Mercifully, there is a breeze: otherwise we would have an apocalypse of insects. Rufus Waddington comes to stay again, as does Maria Whelan, a brilliant pupil, who is to be an angel to me in coming months.

The French cancer Professor haunts me and now makes me vomit. But Maria and Rufus find peppermint growing in the streams, and they make a tea that soothes my stomach. We walk on the hills and pick wild raspberries. Rufus plants garlic in the garden: it grows on the Isle of Wight where he lives. "Why not try it here?" And he makes an enormous kite, seven feet high, from garden canes and plastic: we are amazed that it gets airborne.

Kind Rufus takes me back in the train for the consultation with Dr. Littlewood. Then, in the way of students, he is off to India with Uzbekistan Airlines.

"Do not tell my parents. They think I fly British Airways."

Carmen is at the hospital. If Dr. Littlewood expects a demoralised patient, he gets a dazzling lady who cross-examines him. And there is no aspect of cancer that he is not prepared to analyse. This is hugely different from my first consultants, and the demon French cancer Professor: *do not ever use the word cancer again.*

Carmen probes Dr. Littlewood about treatments that stop short of toxic chemotherapy. There was a trial with interferon in Sweden, she mentions. Dr. Littlewood agrees that interferon is of value but only after chemotherapy when it extends survival. He does not see it as a substitute for chemotherapy. The Swedish patients were in their late sixties, and myeloma progresses more slowly as you get older—and there were only four patients in the trial.

"I wish my students were as bright as you," says Dr. Littlewood to Carmen.

Littlewood knows of Dr. Barlogie and says he will explore any protocol of treatment. Modestly, he does not call himself a total myeloma specialist, but he has treated a number of cases and has a wide experience of leukaemias. His advice to me is unhesitating. Face up. Have chemotherapy. It is not a bogey. Have it soon.

"Suppose I do nothing?"

This was the question I asked in Harley Street.

"You have a seriously compromised immune system. Catch a really bad infection and it could kill you. Also you are at risk from hypercalcaemia."

What of diet?

"As a treatment? You have much too serious a disease."

My impression is that he has not heard of Professor Wynder (*If your friend touches chemotherapy, he's a goner*). As we go on—Dr. Littlewood is unstinting with his time—I ask what will happen to me? He answers in general terms.

I press him to be blunt.

He senses that euphemism would only create anxiety.

"Have the chemotherapy. You will have two years of near normal life. The statistics suggest you may die in the third."

"From the side effects of the treatment?" I ask.

Dr. Littlewood replies that it is false to put it that way since, in his judgement, I could die earlier if I do not have the treatment.

"I can only repeat that with your weakened immune system you may not have the capacity to fight an invasive disease."

I agree to be treated and to start chemotherapy with him on 31 August.

Why do I make this decision? An eminent professor has described Dr. Littlewood to Carmen as having "tremendous art." And I instinctively trust Dr. Littlewood: he is acute, level-headed and kind.

"Are you being influenced by Carmen to have chemotherapy?" asks Rachel.

"Not really."

"Does Christian Carritt know of your decision?"

"Not yet."

"But would you have gone to see Littlewood if Carmen had not found him?"

"I would still be in Scotland."

Rachel and I are driving in the Cotswolds and we stop at a pub. We chat about friends, our favourite paintings and if we will be able to visit Prague, which is our next holiday destination. The thought that we might not makes Rachel cry. I cannot go on to tell her about the French cancer Professor and the fact that he still gives me nightmares. But in Dr. Littlewood's openness and exactness there is such a contrast to the French cancer Professor that to put myself in Littlewood's hands is more than a release, it is an exorcism.

Another factor: just before leaving London David Ambrose rang to say that Wynder (*If your friend touches chemotherapy, he's a goner*) was back in New York and would take my call.

I ring.

"Yuh. Ha. Tosh? How are you doing? Hm? Ambrose. Myeloma. Now, you go see Gonzalez."

Professor Wynder gives me a number, also in New York. I phone Dr. Gonzalez. His office instructs me to listen to a tape that would be mailed at once.

A life in Oxford makes you not oversensitive to the ways of greatness. Why should Professor Wynder waste words on me? None the less, it was a downer. I will go to Dr. Littlewood at the end of the month.

6

The tape comes from Dr. Gonzalez in New York. It is a lecture called *Metabolic Approach to Cancer Therapy* (*metabolic* as in *metabolism,* the process by which food is changed and used by the body).

Dr. Gonzalez begins by telling part of his life story. In 1981 he was doing research in the Department of Pharmacology at Cornell University, an "orthodox" doctor with "very orthodox intentions." A friend asked him to meet Dr. W. D. Kelley, a dentist who tried to cure cancer by nutrition, and was viewed by the medical community as "a piece of sleaze"—Kelley's own words. Dr. Kelley wanted someone to go through his records, which went back twenty-five years. The chairman at Cornell told Gonzalez not to "waste time with a quack." Gonzalez, however, happened to know Dr. Robert Good, President of the Sloan-Kettering Institute, "the most prestigious research centre in the world." Dr. Good took a more favourable view of the project, and Gonzalez spent the summer with Kelley.

In "thousands of cases"—and Gonzalez verified them by contacting patients—he found example after example of people with "appropriately diagnosed cancer, biopsy proven in orthodox institutions, who were alive five and ten years after diagnosis, who should not be alive." In the words of Dr. Gonzalez: "This defied anything I believed possible in medicine."

Dr. Gonzalez decided to select one cancer, and "the worst of cancers," pancreatic. After minute scrutiny, he concluded that Kelley had "the only cases of biopsy proven metastatic pancreatic cancer that apparently had been cured." The patients were alive more than five years later.

Dr. Gonzalez decided to build on Kelley's work. In time "thirty years of stress caught up with Dr. Kelley," who was happy "to pass his ship" to Dr. Gonzalez.

The Kelley/Gonzalez regime has three parts: detoxification, diet and supplements.

"You can't get well if you don't detoxify." Dr. Gonzalez uses coffee enemas. "They are mocked today" but they go back to Florence Nightingale and were a part of orthodox medicine until 1977, "when they became controversial." The enemas work by relaxing muscles in the ducts that lead from the liver to the gall bladder and on to the small intestine. This helps the liver to get rid of toxins. "It is like allowing a dump truck to dump its waste."

Most therapists recommend one diet, usually vegetarian, to everyone. But Dr. Kelley had ten basic diets ranging from vegetarian to all-meat. And there are ninety-five variations on these diets. Everyone had to have their own diet: Kelley went so far as to argue that:

> if something works for a patient, you can be guaranteed it is not going to work for somebody else, and it's going to drive you nuts . . . what you have to do is evaluate what worked in each patient so if you *ever* get a patient like that one, you know what to use as a basis.

The third element, supplements, is viewed in a similar way: "Every protocol has to be individualised, or you are asking for trouble." Also important are "large doses of pancreatic enzymes." Kelley believed that the main defence against cancer was not the immune system, as is widely thought, but the pancreas. This was not his own insight, but it came from an orthodox Scottish doctor, John Beard of the University of Edinburgh, who wrote a book in 1911, *The Enzyme Therapy of Cancer*. Gonzalez argued that this approach had been discarded by the medical profession when Marie Curie discovered radiotherapy. Doctors "literally forgot" about Beard's work.

The tape of Dr. Gonzalez is amazing.

This defied anything I believed possible in medicine.

And Gonzalez expounds his views with relish:

one patient came with his brother who did the talking: "If this therapy was so good how come they're not knocking the doors down to come and see you?" I said, "Well, actually they are knocking the doors to come and see me. It's one of the problems, that's why I don't like to do publicity because I don't want more patients."

The patient's brother then referred to Dr. Kelley:

"I can't let my brother go on a therapy that's developed by a *dentist*"—as he said it he looked like a gorilla whose foot had just been run over by a tractor—"a dirty, filthy dentist."

Gonzalez then imagines a variant of the good cop, bad cop routine. It is the good patient, bad relative:

You know the poor, helpless desperate patient who is so vulnerable because of the disease, and the family loves him and is trying to protect him and help him. Whenever I hear a family member say they're trying to help the patient, I look for the exit.

I am also sent material from the office of Professor Wynder (*If your friend touches chemotherapy, he's a goner*).

ERNST L. WYNDER, MD; D.Sc. h.c.; Dr. med. h.c.
Sloan-Kettering Institute for Cancer Research, New York
1952–1983

TEACHING APPOINTMENTS
Sloan-Kettering, Cornell Medical School: Assistant Professor (1954–1956), Associate Professor (1956–1969) of Preventive Medicine, New York Medical College: Clinical Professor of Community and Preventive Medicine, 1990–present

HOSPITAL APPOINTMENTS
Georgetown University Hospital, Washington, DC: Intern, 1950–1951
Memorial Hospital for Cancer and Allied Diseases, New York, Department of Medicine: 1951–present

AWARDS INCLUDE:
Distinguished Achievement Award, American Society for Preventive Oncology, 1984
Max von Pettenkofer Medal, Munich, Germany, 1988
US Surgeon General's Medal, 1989
Medal of Honor for Clinical Research, American Cancer Society, 1989

Officers Cross of the Order of Merit of the Federal Republic of Germany, 1991

There are also honorary doctorates in the United States
and Germany.

A further paper is headed:

SOME HIGHLIGHTS
OF THE ACCOMPLISHMENTS
OF ERNST L. WYNDER, MD

1. He is generally given credit that his initial study linking
   cigarette smoking and lung cancer, regarded by the
   Journal of the *American Medical Association* (*JAMA*) as a
   landmark article, was not only a crucial work establish-
   ing the causative association between cigarette smoking
   and lung cancer but also presented a key contribution to
   modern epidemiology.
2. His paper on cervical cancer published in 1954 was
   regarded as a landmark article by the World Health
   Organisation (WHO).
3. His ability to attract outstanding colleagues and to organ-
   ize programs in cancer etiology and prevention is exemplified by the American Health Foundation, which he
   founded in 1969 and which today has a staff of about 250.
   The American Health Foundation today is probably the
   best recognized cancer prevention center in the United
   States and receives most of its funding from peer-
   reviewed grants and contracts from the National Cancer
   Institute.

His philosophy is perhaps best embodied in the statement that it should be the function of medicine to help
people die young as late in life as possible.

If Professor Wynder is not the real thing, who is?

I wait for New York time and am given an interview by Dr. Gonzalez's office.

Do I smoke or drink?

Can I see myself taking up to one hundred and fifty supplements a day?

Will I take coffee enemas?

Does my family object to this approach? "We have a lot of trouble with families, Mr. Tosh."

My answers are satisfactory.

Will I get in touch when I am able to come to New York? They wish me good luck.

I wait for California time. I have a friend, Ronny Schwartz, who lives in La Jolla, just north of San Diego. But she also keeps flats in New York and London. She does not know of my cancer, so I fax the news and ask if I might stay in New York when I come to see Dr. Gonzalez.

Ronny phones within minutes. She asks for the details of my diagnosis. Would I tell her more about Dr. Gonzalez?

"Now, Michael, stay put."

In an hour, she sets up a three-way phone consultation with a world authority on myeloma, Professor Syd Salmon of the Cancer Centre at the University of Arizona, Tucson. He interrupts his work to take the call, but his manner gives no suggestion of haste. Our consultation might have been arranged months ago.

"Have you any bone pain?" he asks.

"No."

Good sign. How anaemic am I?

I tell him that my energy seems to be picking up, but that I still rest a good deal.

"So nobody is talking in terms of a blood transfusion?"

Professor Salmon says that it is crucial to start chemotherapy at once. "You have delayed six weeks since diagnosis. Six weeks is the maximum I allow a patient."

He sees no advantage in coming to the States. He knows Dr. Barlogie, whose transcript I read, and thinks highly of him. But there is also Dr. Ray Powles of the Royal Marsden Hospital in Sutton, London. Dr. Powles is excellent and I should go to him at once.

This advice from Professor Salmon is little different from that of my earlier consultants, but I am now a more questioning patient.

"Is there another way of approaching myeloma?" I ask.

"What do you mean?"

I raise nutrition.

Professor Salmon interrupts. He does so courteously: his tone is indistinguishable from how he would explain that he had to adjust a hearing aid.

"Nutrition has no place in the treatment of cancer."

I speak of Dr. Gonzalez. Professor Salmon allows me to finish.

There is an eloquent pause.

"You must not delay starting chemotherapy," he resumes. "Even in six weeks myeloma can progress."

What about Professor Wynder, I ask. Professor Wynder recommended Dr. Gonzalez.

"And where is Wynder?"

I run through the details of Wynder's very distinguished career.

"Ah, in New York," says Salmon. "But he is not a clinician."

This is unexpected and throws me.

"You must not think of travelling," continues Salmon. "Air

pressure is not good for bones. You also have a weakened immune system and could pick up an infection. Powles at the Marsden. Start now. You will be fine with him."

The consultation is at an end.

But Wynder *is* a clinician. I look at his CV. HOSPITAL APPOINTMENTS: Georgetown University Hospital, Washington, DC. Intern, 1950–1951. Memorial Hospital for Cancer and Allied Diseases, New York. Department of Medicine 1951–present.

This makes me angry. Instead of phoning Ronny Schwartz, whom I love, I send a fax to thank her.

Here is her reply:

> *La Jolla, California*
> *14 August*
>
> *Dear Michael,*
>
> *I was so relieved to have your fax! In an hour or so we are leaving for the south of France to help some English friends celebrate their silver wedding. We return the following week. It will be a whirlwind adventure; exhausting but fun, I expect.*
>
> *Dr. Salmon, with whom you spoke on the telephone, was most emphatic that proper treatment, though not a cure, is a controlling factor. At the risk of being a bore, please allow me to repeat what he told me:*
>
> 1) *While not curable, your cancer is* "certainly controllable."
>
> 2) *There is a* "standard treatment" *which is done on an out-patient basis, consisting of two drugs plus predni-zone. This is* not *debilitating.*
>
> 3) *This will control it for a period of perhaps 3–4 years. Following this, there are other treatments to deal with it.*

4) *Such treatment is available in England at the Royal Marsden Hospital in Sutton, where there are specialists.*

5) *Dr. Salmon recommends that you contact Dr. Ray Powles there. It is Ray to whom you turn for advice as to who is best to administer the treatments. You may, of course, use Dr. Salmon's name as reference.*

6) *If you prefer to come to the United States, Dr. Salmon said you could see a Dr. Robert Kyle, or he (Salmon) would be happy to see you himself.*

7) Dr. Salmon urges that you undertake such treatment as soon as possible.

From my own experience, I know that once you have embarked on a course of action and put yourself in the hands of experts, you will feel easier in your mind. You will feel you are waging a battle, determined to win. Indecision is a curse. I have known it under circumstances not dissimilar to yours.

I much look forward to speaking with you when we get back from France.

Love,
Ronny

This will control it for a period of perhaps 3–4 years. But I had read Professor Daniel D. Von Hoff, MD, in one of Carmen's books:

REMEMBER COMPASSION AND QUALITY OF LIFE
It has been well documented that physicians tend to overestimate the survival of their patients by a factor of 3 or 4 times the actual survival of the patient.
Clinical Oncology, p. 90

Following this, there are other treatments to deal with it. But what of Dr. Barlogie?

The secret in terms of long term disease control is not to have a recurrence. Not to have a recurrence. That is the principal law with all cancer. Once the recurrence occurs, the chance to get a cure is minimal. It is going to be shorter and shorter unfortunately.

Is it that Salmon wishes to offer hope?
I do not want illusion.

I am back to square one.

Is it Littlewood and Salmon: treat? Or is it Wynder and Gonzalez: do not treat (but do a lot else)? Christian is away. Who can I turn to?

I must do something. My dreams about the French cancer Professor and the Nazi trains are starting to get worse. I must not go back into that again.

I think of *Cancer and Leukaemia,* the paperback in which I found the breathing exercise. Dr. Jan de Vries went to a lecture . . . yes . . . by no other than Dr. Kelley, the dentist who was the guru of Gonzalez. I read the pages again. Dr. de Vries summarises Kelley's arguments. We all have a unique fingerprint; in the same way each person has a unique metabolism. If this can function better your health will improve. Kelley believed that it may be possible to crack your individual metabolic code, and then boost your glands and organs. If this was done—"to anywhere near 100%"—the body would cure cancer by itself. His aim was to find the perfect food for you, for each individual cancer patient.

Where is Dr. de Vries?

Does he practise? Would he see me?

I ring the publisher of the book and I discover that Dr. de Vries is doing a clinic in North London.

Today.

I phone and I must sound desperate because his secretary says that although there are no cancellations she is sure he will fit me in.

Shawais (who sold me the Mercedes) drives me to the clinic. In the car, I read about the origin of Dr. de Vries's interest in cancer:

> I will never forget seeing my father on his return from the Nazi labour camp. His weight was so low that it seemed as if some skin had been carelessly draped over his bones. My mother did everything within her power to help him regain his health.

Thirty years later, he was found to have cancer:

> Unfortunately, in those days I did not know about the many alternative treatments with which I work nowadays. On operation, the cancer had grown like a climber from the stomach and spread wildly. When I asked the surgeon how long this condition might have been in existence, he answered that it could possibly have been building up to this over the last twenty or thirty years . . . the Nazi regime had possibly claimed another victim.
>
> (*Cancer and Leukaemia*, pp. 29–30)

A restless man moves in and out of the waiting room, smiling and saying hello. He wears an immaculate suit. This is Dr. de Vries. He finds time for me in a crowded schedule.

I describe my cancer.

He writes notes, as if there is not a second to spare, but he scarcely looks at the pad.

His eyes focus on mine.

For a whole minute.

Perhaps more.

I can hear his pen scratching, otherwise we might be anywhere. Then there is a shutdown of his concentration and he writes a prescription.

"One look at you, and you do not need chemotherapy."

I am so surprised that I do not ask why. Dr. de Vries's extra-sensory minute, if it was that, is over. He is recharging his energy for the next patient.

"Potassium drops."

He gives me the prescription, and he stands up.

I cannot let the moment pass. I say that I want to explore the treatment of Dr. Gonzalez, but I have been advised not to travel.

"Brilliant man, Gonzalez. But no need to go to the States. Try my friend Dr. Moolenburgh."

He writes a number in Holland.

I tell him about the Chinese breathing exercise.

"Good. Three times a day. Cancer cells hate oxygen. I learned about the exercise when I was working in a country hospital in China. It may be very ancient."

I cannot impose on more of his time.

"You can sort out this myeloma. Good bye."

I am charged only for the potassium drops, and they are cheap.

Driving back Shawais talks about "extra-sense" doctors in his country, Kurdistan. They can pick up a patient's magnetic field and aura. Perhaps de Vries had this gift. He might have been trained in this mode.

"People are trained?"

"Yes."

I know nothing of Eastern medicine, but I remember an essay by Yeats on an Indian monk, how "the ascetic, if he please, can exhaust in his own body an epidemic that might have swept away the village" (*Essays and Introductions,* p. 433). Such literary style . . . the drama of "exhaust," the idyll of "the village."

But what about "if he please"?

Suppose the monk does not please?

Everyone dies?

De Vries was generous, as in one of my favourite texts: "So let him give, not grudgingly or of necessity, for God loveth a cheerful giver" (2 Corinthians 9:7).

I phone Holland. An answerphone says that Dr. and Mrs. Moolenburgh are away on holiday for some weeks.

August Week 4

I update Christian. She offers to contact Dr. Powles at the Royal Marsden, whom Salmon recommended.

Christian rings back: "Dr. Powles says you have been misinformed. The myeloma treatment is often successful. He can see you tomorrow, but is also happy for you to ring him now."

I phone Dr. Powles. He is extremely approachable and we chat about theatre, politics and Italy. But not medicine. Dr. Powles's motive is to make tomorrow's consultation easier. It is a delightful gesture. We even get on to my view of hope.

"How did you define optimism?" he asks.

"Not my definition, and I am not sure whose it is: an optimist is someone who knows how bad the world is, a pessimist is still finding out."

"We will get on," he laughs.

•   •   •

I tell Rachel that Carmen is to come to the consultation with Dr. Powles.

"Is she always in for the kill?" asks Rachel. But it is wonderful to have a companion, and especially Carmen.

Where Littlewood responded with care to her questions, Powles winds her up. Yet there is no hint of "Hey, I am a world expert and you do not have a basic qualification." If Carmen quotes an article, he evaluates it. They toss about statistics—he is quicksilver with them—predictions, hypothesis, assumptions and interferons. An intrepid lady who takes him on is fun. Also he sees that Carmen is my prop: he is helping me by provoking her to say all she wants, and a bit more.

He is more tough than the other consultants. Am I aware there is a death risk in the treatment? "Always is." But he gives me a 60 per cent chance of complete remission.

"Remission for how long?" asks Carmen.

"What I do is always evolving. I cannot tell."

Has he heard of Gonzalez? No. Wynder? No. Is there anything in a dietary approach? He does not see why it should not complement what he does, but as a substitute? No.

"Suppose I just die of the disease?"

"The zero option is always a possibility."

I give a blood sample but there is to be a further test. "I need to trefine a sample of your bone." Carmen should go to the car.

"Under the cosh," says Powles. A junior doctor and a nurse take me to a small room. I lie on a couch. Local anaesthetic in my side. The nurse holds my hand. Trefining is a process by which a tiny sample is scraped from a bone in the area of the right back hip.

Torture.

•   •   •

Carmen sees that I am furious. Did I dislike Powles?

"No. But I am very sore."

"Anaesthetic wearing off? It is bad stuff. I just refuse to have it."

"What do you do at the dentist?"

"Push my nails into my thumb."

Had this torture not been done on Barlogie's patient? I look up the transcript when I get home.

Yes. With doctorspeak:

Barlogie: It is not going to be very painful, I promise you.

Patient: I had one last week at the Mayo. And it was painful.

Rachel and I are sitting in the garden. Suddenly she says, "Michael, your fury is a world apart from your panic."

Where does this come from?

It is obvious, no doubt, that I am angry, but I have never said a word to Rachel about "panic," about the French cancer Professor or the Nazi trains. But in understanding my state of mind she is bullseye: the French Professor and the trains made me *panic,* my *fury* is a fight back.

Is fury an instinctive antidote to panic, at least to the panic that is either paralysis or directionless activity? Fury is often fury at something, even the search for a target stimulates focus and tactics. Both are counter to disintegration.

We move to a discussion of Christian Carritt and what I call her policy of distraction (Christian has never used the word). You can only distract if there is a basis to distract from. There is no point in distracting someone if the someone has been destroyed. The French Professor's *Do not ever use the word cancer again* drove me mad. If you cannot tell the truth, if you cannot express your deep worries, is not that equivalent to a lobotomy?

As I write, I think of what happened to Ruth Picardie in her final collapse: "it was not to be the lurid paranoia of schizophrenia or the affective excess of mania; it was the blunted, stupid morbidity of the lobotomised."

Blunted and *stupid*.

Please, not for me.

Christian does the opposite. In her quiet way she is giving me time to see what I myself can come up with. Distraction. But I still have nightmares over the French cancer Professor.

Demons never leave quickly, but now I get a surprise.

I start the Chinese breathing exercise.

I do it each day, but familiarity does not make the exercise less daunting. Or time-consuming. You cannot do the exercise, I find, unless you are in the right frame of mind. Dr. de Vries talks about "a few minutes" of relaxed preparation. If only it was a few. Am I too highly strung? It can take an hour before I start.

Breathe in through the toes of the left foot, and up to the hip. Breathe in through the toes of the right foot. Breathe in through the hands.

Breathe in through the base of the spine.

This is more odd than breathing through the toes—and dangerous, or it feels so: if death is likely to come through your spine collapsing, you are conscious that your breath is entering territory to be fought over. It is you versus cancer. All the time you feel about in case there is pain.

Pain is a tumour. If there is no pain, you are over the moon.

Breathe in through the base of the skull. Then the final

vast breath from toes to knees to hips up the spine to neck and through the skull—all breathing in. Then breathe out from the head, all the way down. Both sides together. Seven times.

I start part two of the exercise, visualisation. De Vries recommends that you develop a scenario. I see blood cells coming to a field kitchen for borsch that is made (give them what they do not expect) by a very thin, tall chef. He puts in pigs' knuckles and cuts of rump. There is extra beetroot for the deepest red, and there is contraband salt.

Everyone takes as much as they want.

Igor is in his captain's uniform, an officer to hear any complaints. There is a red flag and a portrait of General Kutuzov, the general who defeated Napoleon on his invasion of Russia. I decided that I could not let into my bloodstream any Second World War generals. To me Stalin is cancer itself.

All the borsch is finished.

The troops are in a good mood and decent to each other. They drink vodka and toast Kutuzov. Skis. Everyone puts on snow uniform. Red troops become white. Killer white cells. We move outside. Sunshields are adjusted.

Breath frosts the air.

We move in quick, silent formations looking for enemies.

A diseased cell is sighted.

It tries to hide.

We accelerate.

Faster!

Keep your eyes skinned.

There it is.

Now.

Attack!

STOP!

AS YOU WERE!

STOI! RAVNYAIS! SMIRNO!

The French cancer Professor, my nightmare, said, *Do not ever use the word cancer again. You influence yourself negatively and make your problem worse.* But I am activating killer cells to attack cancer cells. The killers do not go for unspecified targets. If I am not thinking about cancer, not calling it cancer, if I am not *using the word cancer,* the operation is impossible.

What would the cells attack? If they attacked at random, I would be committing suicide.

It is so obvious.

Why did I not think of it before?

Foutez-moi la paix, mon cher professeur.

However mad the context, this is a breakthrough. And it produces another decision. I am not going to be treated either.

Not now, at any rate.

There is a symbiosis between the French cancer Professor and Dr. Littlewood: remove the demon and you do not need the exorcist.

Wonderful ancient Chinese breathing exercise.

And my dreams, if I have them, are now quiet. I have had two nights of peace. Has Dr. de Vries's "extra sense" also played a part? Did he pierce some inner world in which the Professor made an evil ferment? Whatever, I feel I can climb a mountain.

(As I write, I must emphasise how absurd the symbiosis is with Dr. Littlewood: it was pure coincidence that I met him at this time. It is in no way a reflex of his qualities and kindness. It is the lot of doctors—academics get it too—to be caught in the psychological crossfires of those they try to help.)

•   •   •

A letter comes from Dr. Littlewood:

Dear Michael,

I hope you found the content and outcome of your discussion satisfactory. I think our treatment plan was that you would be treated in Oxford with a protocol C-VAMP and follow this with a high-dose Mephalan protocol and peripheral blood stem cell transplant. This in turn will be followed by interferon.

I enclose photocopies of appropriate pages showing you details of the chemotherapy that you will be following.

I am sorry I forgot to mention to you that the best way of administering this chemotherapy is through a Hickman line which can be placed into one of the big veins (the superior vena cavae) and tunnelled out under the skin of your chest wall. This then stays in place for the duration of your treatment.

If you are agreeable I can arrange this for Wednesday, 31st August, and you should then be able to start treatment later then the same day.

Dr. T. J. Littlewood
Consultant Haematologist

This is a kind and responsible letter, but in my current state of mind Dr. Littlewood's *I forgot to mention* hits a nerve. Who can blame Dr. Littlewood if he forgot things during a session with Carmen as well as me? But his phrase *I forgot to mention* makes me paranoid about gradual disclosure, about bad news dripping out. Will there be more? And I saw a Hickman line at the Marsden: a patient's shirt was open and a rubber tube hung from his chest.

"They get infected easily," said Carmen, "so there is a danger of septicaemia, which can be fatal."

Even without the septicaemia—which, I am sure, is

rare—the Hickman line struck me as eerie: I thought it came from the world of Mrs. P. and opportunistic pneumonia, where even after treatment you need prophylactic sprays. Forget the spray and the germs kill you.

Also my mother explodes at the idea of the Hickman line. She is phoning from Scotland but she pictures it like a horror movie. I write to Dr. Littlewood and decline his offer of treatment.

28 AUGUST—3 SEPTEMBER

"How are you getting on with the juicer?" asks Rachel.

"Juicer?"

"Darling, the girl sent you a juicer."

"No."

"Carmen did."

"You have got it wrong."

"For God's sake, Michael, do you bother to read her letters?"

Rachel finds one that came a month ago:

31 July

Dear Michael,

Here are some odds and ends for you. The vitamins I would check out with one of your doctors, as with myeloma I imagine, one has to be careful not to overload possibly overtaxed kidneys.

I am a fan of the enclosed book, Leslie Kenton, Raw Energy, *which has a lot to say on cancer diets. I am tracking down Max Gerson,* Cancer Therapy, *which seems to be the seminal work. But you could certainly follow the* Raw Energy *precepts.*

Incidentally, I have a juicer I am not using. Shall I send it to you? Where?

I will also send Linus Pauling's book on vitamin C, as soon as I have it. If you do decide to try mega-doses of vitamin C, you should note that Pauling thinks it very important to build up to a high dose slowly, maybe over a week or more, and not *stop abruptly.*

Taper it out.

In fact, why stop it at all . . . it is also best in split doses, say 3 or 4 a day.

Love,
Carmen.

Rachel makes me ashamed to have taken so little notice of Carmen, and we start to read the book in the parcel. Leslie Kenton is as respected a writer in her field as you can find. Her book, *Raw Energy*, starts with a foreword by Dr. Malcolm Carruthers MRC Path., MD, MRCGP.

Leslie Kenton is not a doctor, and Rachel reminds me that Carmen once described herself as an "amateur hypochondriac." Rachel insists that we begin with Dr. Carruthers:

Healthy eating is a timeless science, researched for thousands of years in different civilisations but surprisingly neglected this century. Here we are given the full history of the use of raw food diet in what ancient Taoist tradition considered the goal of life—achieving harmony. Streams of thought in religious, philosophical and medical teaching have given rise to many different ideas for balancing the opposing aspects of human life. To some they represent the dynamic, often destructive, male principle seen against the constant nurturing female principle, the shiva versus shakti of Indian philosophies, yang versus yin of Chinese traditions. Modern scientists would see them as catabolic and anabolic, acid or alkaline producing metabolic processes, and sympathetic fight and flight or para-sympathetic rest and digest divisions of the autonomic or automatic nervous system preparing the body for war or peace.

As the theoretical physicist Fritjof Capra describes in his recent book *The Turning Point,* we are now beginning to appreciate the urgency of the need to move towards a more balanced mid-point between these polarities if we are to avoid disaster at both the individual and global level.

"Is it a new form," Rachel asks, "a literary genre?"

We call it the medical overture. There is expectation, a sense of brio, huge vistas of history and thought, East and West, digestion and apocalypse.

"Who but these idiots," says Rachel, "would write *sympathetic fight and flight or para-sympathetic rest and digest divisions of the autonomic or automatic nervous system?*"

Leslie Kenton herself is different. Her prose is lucid and she argues that a diet 75 per cent raw food has great benefits: "the Germans and the Swedes and the Swiss have for generations catalogued the healing effects of a diet high in fresh raw vegetables and fruits (*Raw Energy,* p. 13)." "The diseases which are healed," Kenton continues, include "long term crippling" diseases "such as arthritis and cancer."

"Do not get overexcited," says Rachel. "An old friend is in the slime, the Catch-22. Ms. Kenton writes: 'No book can replace adequate medical care. We would suggest that any reader who is unwell seek the attention and care of a nutritionally aware physician' [p. 14]. But Dr. Carruthers MRC Path., MD, MRCGP says: 'Nutritionally aware physicians are few and far between, especially when it comes to factors such as the subtle energies of living plants and plant enzymes which are . . . covered by the Kentons' [p. 10]. Result? When you need a physician, none can be found."

•　　•　　•

Rachel plans to stay with friends in Wiltshire and I am to go to Scotland. But I will have to travel alone, and my car is up north.

Can I face the train?

I am not having bad dreams, but has the French cancer Professor really gone? Will a train bring him back? I am scared. I decide to travel in a sleeper so that I can lie down and do the Chinese breathing exercise.

All night if necessary.

I go to London and meet Benjamin. We eat at a Lebanese restaurant. Not much conversation, except that he does not think it coincidence that we should both be in a black period at the same time.

Euston Station. The train journey starts and I begin the routines.

Toes.

Hands.

I rest between each section. No hurry when there is all night. Spine. Skull. Visualisation.

Borsch. Lavish. The soldiers hunted boar. Igor regards boar as German and he relishes any hint of retaliation for the Second World War. (Russia is probably full of boar, but this is visualisation, not logic.) The troops smoke. Igor lies on his tent mat, the same that he brought to London.

Skis.

Vodka.

Toasts.

"Kutuzov! To victory! To our little father!"

"Za Kutuzova! Za pobiedu! Za nashego batiushku!"

Suddenly General Kutuzov glares and steps down from his portrait.

"This is wonderful," shout the troops. "Eto tchudo!"

Everyone cheers.

Kutuzov takes the leather strap off his blind eye. The blind eye goes bloodshot.

"Watch out!" shouts a soldier, "Do not punish us: Nie veli kaznit!"

"Lead us to battle!" cries Igor.

"Viedi nas!" shout the troops.

They line up. Kutuzov marches through. He puts on skis. We all put on snow combats.

We hunt.

We spot the French cancer Professor from the Nazi trains.

He tries to hide. The troops flush him out. He hides again.

Now Kutuzov leads the chase.

Down a slope.

Down another.

Into a music hall, where ventriloquists are training dummies to say "cancer." This is in Ostende.

We go to a restaurant, and have a supper of langoustines. (How it happened.)

Not the end of the French Professor, probably, but I can lie on the bunk and listen to the train.

Benjamin. If our misfortunes are more than coincidence, his is worse than mine.

I have brought a book about the Czar under whom Kutuzov served, Alexander I. I read how Alexander was brought up by the Empress Catherine the Great. One of her ideas was to make the boy sleep near cannons that were fired for reveille each day. She wished Alexander to be brave, but she only made him deaf.

I remember that the painter Renoir protected his children against noise "especially gunfire, asserting that it harmed the child's delicate sense of hearing" (Jean Renoir, *Renoir My Father,* p. 281).

The artist versus power.

I take out Leslie Kenton's *Raw Energy,* the book I started to read with Rachel.

Physician, heal thyself, Kenton writes:

> Many physicians and healers have cured themselves of serious illness by eating uncooked foods. As a last resort Danish physician Kristine Nolfi turned to raw foods in an effort to beat breast cancer. She won. Then she taught her patients about this natural form of healing. Her success was so great (as was the fury her treatments unleashed among her orthodox peers).

I imagine Rachel on *the fury among orthodox peers . . .*

> Her success was so great (as was the fury her treatments unleashed among her orthodox peers) that she gave up using drugs altogether and started the Humlegaarden sanatorium in Denmark . . .
>
> The American expert on raw juice therapy Dr. Norman W. Walker, now 107, rid himself of the excruciating pains of neuritis with raw foods . . .

Jolly dog, Dr. Norman Walker.

> Live raw fruit and vegetable juices are an essential part of anti-cancer diets. Raw juices do most of the excellent

things that solid raw foods do but in a way which places the minimum strain on the digestive system.

My stomach now needs all the help it can get.

The concentrated vitamins, minerals, trace elements, enzymes, sugars and proteins they contain, are absorbed into the bloodstream almost as soon as they reach the stomach and small intestine . . .

Memo: I must get that juicer from Carmen.

Of course huge quantities of fresh fruit and vegetables are needed to produce juice by crushing or centrifuging.

My friends Hugh and Catherine Bell, who run the Health Food Centre in Carlisle, will have to help, and I shall be begging my old friend and neighbour Jimmy Hewitson to make deliveries.

The Gerson cancer diet, for example, which prescribes ten 8 oz glasses a day of fresh carrot, apple and green vegetable juices, uses some 1800 lb/820 kg carrots a year, 125 lb/57 kg green peppers, 145 cabbages and upwards of 1300 oranges.

One hundred and forty-five cabbages? I might as well be in Russia. Except where would I find the oranges?

When I get to my house in Scotland, I remember that I bought a vegetable juicer some years ago. There was a mad spell of juicing—Benjamin, who was staying, called it "gut busting"—and we then gave up.

I find the machine in the attic.

Maria Whelan helps me make juices of apple and carrot; apple, carrot and beetroot; even apple and nettle, to which I become addicted.

And we need mammoth quantities.

7

I go back to London and stay with my wonderful friend Olga Polizzi.

She urges me to see a Vietnamese doctor. He does not want me to reveal his name and I shall call him Dr. H.

"As it is," he says, "I can scarcely make time for the friends you send me."

Dr. H. qualified as an orthodox doctor under the French in Vietnam and was head of an army surgical unit during the war against the North. After the communist victory, he was put in a concentration camp.

He was released.

"They found they needed doctors, and those from South were better qualified."

Dr. H. decided to flee Vietnam. He came to the UK and qualified again as an orthodox doctor. But he now practises acupuncture.

"How does acupuncture work?" I ask Dr. H. when he goes through my symptoms.

"We do not understand much. I cannot cure your cancer; I try to help your body fight it."

I lie on a couch. Dr. H. puts needles above my ankles, in

my legs, my stomach and my hands. I then rest for an hour. When I get home, I sleep very deeply.

Carmen decides to run a medifind search on myeloma. She finds that a Professor Sherman in New York has written about the use of interferon in myeloma in *Proceedings of the American Society of Clinical Oncology*.

Carmen phones Professor Sherman, who takes her call. In the course of a long chat, Carmen makes a discovery: Professor Sherman has a myeloma patient whom he has not treated with either chemotherapy or interferon, and whose disease has remained static for ten years.

Only one patient, but for us it is a breakthrough.

Up to now our thinking has been in the shadow of the book I read in St. Catherine's library on the day I was diagnosed, four months ago:

> Multiple myeloma is incurable. The median survival time from clinical confirmation to death is under a year in untreated patients, and two to three years with treatment. Some 15% die within the first three months.

Carmen writes to thank Professor Sherman:

September 5

Dear Dr. Sherman,

The mark of an excellent physician is, to me, restraint. So I write to thank you for your good counsel to me concerning my friend, Michael Gearin-Tosh, who was recently diagnosed as having myeloma.

It was extremely generous of you to speak at such length to an unknown and unexpected caller. This is really deeply appreci-

ated, in particular because you have provided the first profes-sional confirmation of the possible value of delaying treatment—which both my friend and I feel must be intuitively right. Michael will certainly come and see you if he does decide to go over and canvas American medical opinion.

In the meantime we will be doing some monitoring. But not exactly doing nothing. Michael has been taking vitamin C, follows a strict diet and has started juicing vegetables. We are exploring the Max Gerson cancer therapy which you may know, and the Linus Pauling, Abram Hoffer recommendations for vitamin supplements. There now seems to be some concrete evidence that the Pauling/Hoffer vitamin regimen has extended the lives of terminal cancer patients significantly and in a small percentage promoted "cures." So one assumes at an early stage in cancer, it must hold more promise. (I can send you the references if you are interested.)

I still wonder whether in such a holistic approach, interferon might not have something to add. And if you do know of any-one testing in further, please let me know. I gather much is still to be discovered about the clinical uses of cytokines.

I enclose Michael's results since diagnosis. You may care to comment if it is indeed wise to hold off until another set of tests, say in October.

As your time and expertise are valuable, please do not hesi-tate to bill me.

We would value your comments without holding you responsible for our future actions . . .

Once again, many thanks!

Kind regards,
Carmen Wheatley

SEPTEMBER WEEK 2

At my next acupuncture session, I tell Dr. H. how excited I am about Professor Sherman's survivor.

Dr. H.'s face does a double take: mouth joyous like a child, eyes satiric.

"Am I wrong to be pleased?" I ask.

"Maybe your number not up."

Dr. H. puts in needles and points to the roof.

"Typhoon when I escape Vietnam. My number not up." Dr. H. tells me that he was in a crowded boat. A typhoon tore off the rudder and they drifted for three days until a ship from Glasgow came by.

"We always send cards to the captain."

Dr. H.'s wife, a Vietnamese beauty, runs his office.

As I pay, I mention Dr. H.'s escape.

"I was there too."

"In the boat?"

"Yes. And three children. Whole family."

"How big was the boat?"

"Five metres wide, ten metres long."

"How many people?"

"Two hundred and forty-six."

"Did you have water?"

"We lost it in the typhoon. And food."

"You had nothing?"

"No food, no water, three days. And nights."

"Was it hot?"

"Yes."

"Were there sharks?"

"I did not ask."

• • •

I am so humbled by their courage that I cannot do the Chinese exercise when I get home.

Carmen rings. She has found a doctor in London who put himself on the Gerson therapy, and he is happy to see me this afternoon.

"But Carmen, I must know something about the Gerson therapy."

"Read Kenton. I sent it to you."

"I am reading it, but I have not come to Gerson yet."

"Anyway . . ." Carmen breaks off and giggles.

"What is the joke?" I ask.

"Kenton misses something out, Michael."

"Yes?"

"Coffee enemas."

"Coffee enemas . . . do I remember Dr. Gonzalez talking about them on his tape?"

"Oh yes. Gonzalez. And Florence Nightingale. The soldiers in the Crimea got them."

"I have never had an enema."

"Lucky you, Michael. The Gerson therapy enema is two pints."

"Of coffee?"

"Yes."

"You mean two milk bottles . . . of coffee . . ."

"And every day. Four times."

"Two pints four times?"

"Correct."

"That is a gallon."

"And I have found out something else."

"Enough for today."

"Do you know who was Rachel's co-examiner when I applied for Oxford? Before you took me?"

"No idea."

"There was an examiner in Modern Languages at Rachel's college, Joan Spencer."

"I know Joan. She is delightful."

"She has had cancer. And cured it with Gerson. Go on, phone her up about enemas."

Joan Spencer is much loved by two of my closest friends, Derek and Margaret Davies, and I have had the pleasure of meeting her for many years.

I phone.

"Joan, I never knew you had cancer."

"Yes, years ago."

In 1983 a black mole was found on Joan's arm. Was it melanoma, the dreaded skin cancer? "Yes," said a specialist after surgery. "No," said a second. A third thought there had been malignancy, but it had gone.

In 1987 a lump appeared on Joan's armpit. It was found to be a highly malignant metastasised melanoma, and it was removed by surgery. Joan read a book by Beata Bishop about curing melanoma, and this led her to do the Gerson therapy.

She remains free of cancer today.

"Do you remember Carmen Wheatley?" I ask.

"Yes. Very beautiful girl. Blonde hair. Had to sort her out. Did she not end up with you?"

"She is interesting me in Gerson."

"Have you got cancer?"

"Yes."

"For God's sake, do not let the doctors kill you."

"Carmen suggested that I ask you about coffee enemas."
"Delightful. I read *War and Peace* having mine."

Joan tells me that the place to buy enema equipment is a health store in Paddington Street.

I go at once.

"Tubes or bucket, sir?"

I do not know.

"There are tube enemas, sir, and buckets. Different process. For yourself, is it?"

He speaks softly, but the shop goes still.

"Sara, have we a tube?"

They unpack an object made of pink rubber.

"The problem is?"

I quickly say that I do not see how two pints of coffee can fit into the balloon at the end of the tube.

"Two pints? Sara, he needs the bucket."

The Gerson doctor is Dr. Bernard Courteney Mayers. He lives in an enchanting house on Brook Green.

"The garden was a help during the therapy. And two years will pass. Not so long, you know."

(Two years is the minimum time for the therapy.)

Dr. Courteney Mayers urges me to go to the Gerson clinic in Mexico.

"You will start off in optimal conditions. Stay a month or two if you can afford it."

"Has the therapy worked for you?" I ask.

"No recurrence so far."

"Are the enemas crucial?"

"Essential. Four. Every day."

"How does one actually . . ."

Bernard looks out a plastic bucket. Simple procedure: coffee at blood heat, lubricant guess where, lie down, insert, open a valve (reach for *War and Peace*), fifteen minutes later sit on the loo.

"How will you do for injections?"

I have not read that Gerson patients inject with a mixture of liver juice and vitamin B_{12}.

"It is a big injection," says Bernard, and fits up a demonstration syringe. "Be sure to keep it straight and go for the buttock here": he does an athletic twist.

I am terrified of injections, and my face tells all.

"Or you could find a nurse," says Bernard. "To start with."

The Chinese breathing exercises are still flat.

I get through the routines of the first part, but the visualisations do not work.

As soon as my mind relaxes what surfaces is Dr. H. and his family escaping from Vietnam, and the grace of Benjamin in thinking of me in his terrible sorrow.

8

I mention the Gerson therapy to David Ambrose, who says he will check it out with Professor Wynder.

David rings back.

"Wynder knows all about it. Gerson died in 1958."

"Old hat?"

"Not how he put it."

"At least Gerson did not go in for chemotherapy."

"No."

"So the therapy is okay?"

"No."

"Why?"

"Wynder just said, 'I would not put my dog on Gerson.' "

My mother's cocker spaniels are champions in many countries. She judges Crufts. I was brought up with dogs, seldom less than fifty and often more.

Our dogs were kept outside. They would work for hours on heather moors, and I knew each dog by name, I would sometimes sit up at nights when a mother was in labour.

I once saw a champion on a bleak Perthshire hill stalk a hare.

So in canine matters I am a match for Professor Wynder.
A dog of his would be overweight and snappy.

I force myself, as I do every day, to start the breathing exercise.

Toes.

In. Out.

Seven times.

Other foot.

Seven times.

Blast Wynder.

Is it my ill luck, when I find a way forward, to be
squashed?

Breathe through the fingers.

In. Out.

Other hand.

Spine.

Skull.

Please, visualisation, work. Here is my Russian kitchen.
Try to smell the borsch.

New idea.

Perhaps the chef brings in a slovenly poodle. Wynder's
dog.

But we are interrupted by the phone.

It is Carmen.

"Michael, I rang the Bristol Cancer Help Centre and
asked them about Gerson."

"Yes?"

"The voice on the phone said, 'We do not do Gerson. It
is too stressful.' I asked the voice, 'Don't you think death by
cancer is stressful?' End of conversation."

"They rang off?"

"More or less."

"Snappy."

"So I phoned Charlotte Gerson. Daughter of the great man."

"Carmen, wow."

"She runs the Gerson clinic in Mexico. Some lady."

"Look who is talking."

"Michael, I am a pigmy compared with Charlotte Gerson. First, she tells me off for wasting money because I left too long a message on her answerphone—and she is ringing from California to scold me. It could have been Rachel dusting me down."

"Not quite."

"As you know, I am doubtful about the enemas."

"I did not know."

"Coffee is noxious, and they sound so disgusting. I quiz Charlotte Gerson. Or try to. 'Your friend must understand,' she says, 'and you should too, that every element in the therapy is there for a purpose. Do it all. Ask later.' "

"You are sure you were not annoying Charlotte Gerson?"

"I went on to ask if she has success with myeloma patients. 'They have all been weakened by chemotherapy and radiation before coming, but I see no reason why the therapy should not work.' "

"I see."

"Could be worse."

"Yes."

"You seem low, Michael. Anything wrong?"

"I have just had Wynder on the topic of Gerson. He told David Ambrose he would not put his dog on it."

"Would not put his dog on it?"

"What the man said."

"But does his dog have cancer?"

"Do dogs get cancer?"

"Yes. But, of course, that would not have been his point."

"No."

"By the way," Carmen continues, "Charlotte Gerson has a friend in Oxford."

"Who?"

"Guess."

"No idea."

"Joan Spencer. And did Joan go to Mexico to the Gerson clinic? No. She did the therapy all by herself."

"Good for her."

"Yes it is. She did it all herself. So you can too."

"What is Carmen playing at?" asks Rachel. "One moment you are off to another consultant, next moment she has you scrubbing carrots."

"She is looking at various options."

"Looking at options is fine if she were giving you a tutorial. But you have cancer. It is role reversal gone mad. Why do you put up with it?"

"There is a cancer therapy she is finding out about. The Gerson therapy. Joan Spencer did it."

"Joan had cancer?"

"Yes."

"I never knew. Joan is a good scholar and sound woman. She tried carrots?"

"Yes."

"Carrots cure cancer?"

"The juice seems to help."

"So why does not everyone do it?"

•   •   •

The breathing exercise is difficult.

Even the first part takes more time: I have to relax for so long before I can start.

Going through the body bone by bone makes you identify with each part, as it were come to terms with it.

The visualisations have a life of their own.

They will not be forced.

Wynder's dog is not accepted as part of the scenario.

I had hoped that Kutuzov might clip it.

But now even the borsch kitchen is nothing.

The most I can manage is a hunt after cancer cells, and the only hunter is me.

I go through tunnels, not ski on mountains.

I buy Dr. Gerson's book, *A Cancer Therapy*. It is a summary of thirty years' clinical practice and, although written for doctors, Gerson believed that "intelligent laymen" could understand "the main problems."

Not easy.

At least not at first sight.

Even Rachel is daunted by the prospect of two hundred and fifty pages of theory and comment, then fifty case histories with X-rays and photographs.

"The X-rays are nightmares," she says.

I spot an appendix in the book. It contains a short lecture by Gerson.

He was seventy-five when he gave the lecture, "and still," he argues, "I am convinced that cancer does not need a specific treatment" (*A Cancer Therapy*, p. 406).

This is an extraordinary statement.

Stand back from it.

No specific treatment for cancer?

I tell Rachel that at the Royal Marsden Hospital there was shelf after shelf of medical journals, thick volumes called *Myeloma, Proceedings of the American Society of Clinical Oncology, Journal of Clinical Pathology, Diagnostic Radiology, Acta Haematologica, Scandinavian Journal of Haematology, Journal of Interferon and Cytokine Research, Japanese Journal of Clinical Oncology.*

Yet Gerson thought that cancer *does not need a specific treatment*?

"What can the man mean?" says Rachel.

In the lecture, Dr. Gerson tells how he came upon his therapy.

As a young man he suffered from severe migraines. Doctors told him that there was no cure. But Gerson found that by changing his diet the migraines came less often. He cut out salt, pickled and smoked food and most fats; he also ate more fresh fruit and vegetables.

When Gerson qualified as a doctor he recommended this diet to his patients. Then he was told that the diet cured the friend of a patient who had *lupus vulgaris* or skin tuberculosis.

Gerson described the next step as "funny." Another way of describing it is that he encountered a lady of great character.

"She is just like you," I say to Rachel, as we read. Charlotte Gerson in another guise, might have been Carmen's comment.

Dr. Gerson wrote:

When I was a physician for internal diseases in Bielefeld [Germany] in 1928, I was called to see a lady. She told me she was operated on in a big clinic nearby, and they found a cancer of the bile duct.

I saw the operation scar.

She was running a high fever, was jaundiced. I told her, "Sorry, I can do nothing for you. I don't know how to treat cancer. I have not seen results, especially in such an advanced case where there is no longer the possibility of operation."

But she said, "No, doctor, I called you because I saw the results in your treatment of tuberculosis and arthritis [also by Gerson's diet] in various cases. Now, here is a pad and you write down a treatment.

"Also on that table over there, there is a book, and in that book, you will be good enough to read to me aloud the chapter called *The Healing of Cancer.*"

Dr. Gerson did as he was told, walked to the table and fetched the volume:

It was a big book of about 1200 pages on folk medicine and in the middle there was that chapter.

I started to read.

That book was edited by three school teachers . . . None of them practised medicine.

"Dr.ink to that!" says Rachel. "Real school teachers who care for life and think for themselves."

She pours a whisky.

"Long may teachers survive, backbone of the community!"

"Cheers!"

"Michael, when did the ladies write the book?"

"I am not sure the school teachers were female. It just says 'three school teachers.' "

Dr. Gerson read the chapter to the sick lady:

In it there was something about Hippocrates who gave these patients a special soup. I should like to tell you, we use that soup at the present time! That soup from that book, out of the practice of Hippocrates—550 years before Christ! He was the greatest physician at that time, and I even think the greatest physician of all time. He had the idea that the patient has to be detoxified with the soup and with some enemas and so on.

I read and read but finally I told the lady, "Look, because of my tuberculosis treatment physicians are opposed to me. Therefore I'd like not to treat you."

"Yes, yes," says Rachel. "*Physicians are opposed to me.* What do you expect."

I tell her about the case of the Danish doctor in Kenton's book, the doctor who cured her own breast cancer with raw food and "unleashed fury among her orthodox peers."

"Damn them," growls Rachel, and pours more whisky.

We go back to Gerson's lecture:

Again the lady insisted, "I'll give you in writing that you are not responsible for the outcome of the treatment and that I insisted that you do so." So with that signed statement, I thought, all right, let's try.

"Darling, you mean that Dr. Gerson, a fully qualified doctor and from the University of Berlin, felt he had to get a *signed statement*? Heavens above. And the poor lady who was ill: was it Molière who wrote that you have to die according to the rules?"

Gerson continued:

I wrote down the treatment. It was almost the same which I used for tuberculosis patients at the University Clinic in Munich with Professor Sauerbruch.

It is always written in scientific books that tuberculosis and cancer are both degenerative diseases where the body has to be detoxified. I tried—and the patient was cured!

Six months later she was up and around in the best condition.

Then she sent me two other cancer cases.

One of her family with a stomach cancer where it had been found during an attempted operation that there were metastasised glands around the stomach—also cured!

And I had to cure then, against my will, a third case.

"Against his will?" asks Rachel. "A doctor saving life *against his will?"*

"Gerson gives the reason, and it will not surprise you: 'I expected to have still more opposition from the medical profession.'"

"Michael," says Rachel, "if your preoccupation with Russia and Chekhov did not make you so indifferent to Shaw, you would remember what I read from *The Doctor's Dilemma*: 'The medical profession is a murderous absurdity.'"

"Now, now."

"Doctors murder each other."

"Rachel . . ."

"Murder. They do. As a fact. Of course they kill patients, but they murder each other as well."

She marches out, and I finish Gerson's lecture:

The third case was also a stomach cancer. It was also cured. Three cases were tried and all three cases were cured!

I have to tell you that up to this day, I don't know how this happened, how I stumbled into it, how this was achieved.

(*A Cancer Therapy*, pp. 403–4)

Rachel comes back with *Encyclopaedia Britannica*, the grand old Cambridge edition of 1913.

"Paracelsus. Great pioneering physician killed by other doctors," she declares.

"Physically?"

"Yes. Murder. The cause of the death of Paracelsus is uncertain, says the *Encyclopaedia*, but it is likely that 'he was thrown down a steep place by some emissaries of the physicians.' *Emissaries* . . . fine word. Mafia has soldiers, doctors have to have emissaries. Typical jargon. Anyway, it is murder."

"Appears so."

"What do you mean, 'appears'? Doctors are a quarrelsome, vicious lot, and always have been. Do you know they persecuted Galen? His colleagues drove him out of Rome. Too successful at cures."

There is drama in medicine, if only it was not for real.

September Week 4

I tell Dr. H. about the Gerson therapy.

"But it is not specific to cancer," I say.

"Do not worry if not specific. Are your breathing exercises specific?"

"No."

"May be a good thing."

"Why?"

"Western medicine has wonderful diagnostic tools. Here,

in UK, you test the heart, bone density, whatever. But in Vietnam we had no such tools. In one or two hospitals, perhaps, but in the country . . . so what can we do for the poor people?"

"Must be very difficult."

"The monks learn acupuncture. From the head monk. He pass on from monks before. And the young monks watch. Poor people come to the temples. They are treated. Acupuncture. For free."

As a character says in Chekhov, "I came looking for prose and walk slap into poetry" (Borkin in *Ivanov*, Act III).

A letter comes from Moscow:

> *Dear Michael!*
>
> *How are you? I'm fine. I could not write you before, because I went in the Caucasus to my parents.*
>
> *My dear friend, I want to tell you* thank you very much. *It was very nice time in my life. I can forget it never. Write me about your next visit to Moscow or S. Petersburg. Can you go to Moscow? I'll be happy if you stay in my flat. Please, forgive me, when I was wrong sometimes.*
>
> *How is your health? I went to the church. I'll be to go every week. I try to give money beggars. I'll ask a priest to offer prayers for you.*
>
> *OK? Michael! Think about your health more. I'm working now. I'm cold. I cannot forget a time from 16.07 to 29.07.*
>
> *Take care! Moscow.*
>
> *Igor.*

Is it the letter from Igor? The idea of the Russian beggars?

(Igor saw me give money in Moscow, but we never discussed it.)

Is it the thought of the monks treating the poor in Vietnam?

Is it the determined lady in Dr. Gerson's book?

Benjamin phones, and we chat about nothing for ten minutes. Is it that?

Whatever.

The breathing exercises suddenly become easy. I get into them quickly: only five minutes or so relaxing before I start.

Toes.

Hands.

Spine.

I find it strenuous when I have to imagine breath going up the spine and crossing the lungs: there is a time of anatomical struggle.

Head.

Total journey from toes to skull, again with the struggle of crossover.

My visualisations change. There is no carnival, no kitchen, no Russian troops, no Kutuzov. I race down tunnels, which seem to be veins. But there is a new feature. I have unidentified friends who help me. Together, we spot cancer cells and we fight them.

I read more in Gerson's book. The story of how he developed his therapy becomes interwoven with escape from the Nazis. After leaving Germany for Vienna, Gerson writes:

> I could no longer separate myself from the problem of cancer. In Vienna I tried six cases and in all six cases, no results—all failures. That was shocking.
>
> The sanatorium where I treated my patients was not so

well organized for dietary treatments. They treated other diseases by other methods and didn't pay much attention to diet. So, I attributed the failures to that.

Then Gerson was forced to flee to Paris. He tried seven cases of cancer. Four failed, but three were cured. The case of a lady from Armenia especially interested him:

I had to work against the whole family. There were many physicians in the family, and I had plenty of trouble.

But, anyway, I came through in that case. She had cancer of breast which re-grew. Every time the family insisted that she was "so much down." She weighed only 78 pounds. She was skin and bones and they wanted me to give her egg yolks.

I gave her small amounts of egg yolks—the cancer re-grew.

Then they insisted that I give her meat, raw chopped meat.

I gave her this and the cancer re-grew.

The third time, they wanted me to give her some oil. I gave her the oil and the third time the cancer re-grew.

But, anyway, three times I could eliminate the cancer again and cure.

And still I had no idea what cancer was.

If somebody asked me about the theory, just what it was I was doing, I had to answer, "I don't really know myself."

The Nazis then drove Gerson to the States:

I couldn't get the cancer problem and the cure of the first three cases out of my mind. I kept thinking, "It must be possible, it would be a crime not to do it."

• • •

The Gerson book is so interesting that I press David Ambrose to get more out of Wynder (*I would not put my dog on Gerson*).

The result is a fax from Wynder's office not about Gerson but about Dr. Gonzalez.

An insurance company, the Mutual Benefit Life of Kansas, Missouri, spent several months meeting patients of Dr. Gonzalez and examining case histories:

> The results are indeed extraordinary. We have seen excellent outcomes with a pancreatic cancer case (metastatic to the liver) diagnosed at Mayo clinic. We have seen return to work for over two years in a case of metastatic melanoma previously operated on twice (unsuccessfully) at Memorial Sloan-Kettering. We have seen long-term survival in terminal lung cancers . . .

And so it went on. Cancer type after cancer type.

The report concluded that "the approach is so unorthodox that although a lot of doctors in academic medicine now refer patients to Dr. Gonzalez, no one is pressing for research into his methods."

To be *unorthodox* is one thing.

But to have an insurance company, a factual, meticulous, dry and calculating institution in favour of an unorthodox approach . . .

Surely, this is significant.

Carmen comes to Oxford and we hold a council of war.

We decide that I must go to Gonzalez.

Carmen writes to him:

September 23 1994

Dear Dr. Gonzalez,

I am writing to you on behalf of Michael Gearin-Tosh of St. Catherine's College, Oxford. You were highly recommended to him by Dr. Ernst L. Wynder, and you will have some details already, as Michael has had a preliminary phone conversation with your secretary, Bridget, in August.

Michael was diagnosed as having multiple myeloma, 1gG Lambda, Stage 1, in late June. His oncologist is Dr. Ray Powles of the Royal Marsden Hospital, Surrey. Because Michael's prognostic factors are currently good, we have all jointly decided simply to monitor him for the time being. (See attached summary of results of tests at the Marsden on 23.8.94.) This being the case, I have strongly urged him to follow a gentle, alternative therapy in the meantime . . .

We listened to your tape with great interest, but would like some more specific information on your treatment therapy. Please can you tell us whether Kelley's One Answer to Cancer *is still available, and if so, where?*

Secondly, and more importantly, as Dr. Wynder clearly thinks you have one of the best "alternative" therapies available, we would like the answers to the following questions:

1) How many multiple myeloma cases have you treated and with what success?

2) What is the rationale *for your treatment of multiple myeloma?*

I know you are a very busy man, but we would greatly appreciate answers to the above. Michael would be very happy also to pay your standard fee for a preliminary phone consultation—via myself—in particular as both his oncologist and I have strongly advised him against foreign travel, on account of his great susceptibility to infection. (It was a very nasty viral pneu-

monia which led to his diagnosis in June.) We will be glad to provide any other information you might require.

Yours sincerely
Carmen Wheatley

NICHOLAS J. GONZALEZ, MD

September 23, 1994

Dear Dr. Carmen Wheatley:
Thank you for your recent fax. However, having reviewed this as well as the previous information given our office by Mr. Gearin-Tosh, I do not think it best he pursue this approach.
I appreciate your interest in my work.

Sincerely,
Nicholas J. Gonzalez, MD

I do not want to give up.

Carmen writes again and Dr. Gonzalez replies at more length:

NICHOLAS J. GONZALEZ, MD

September 26, 1994

Dear Dr. Wheatley:
I appreciate your fax regarding Mr. Gearin-Tosh. I did not mean to imply that he would not benefit from my therapy, as I have many patients with myeloma who are doing very well. The problem with Mr. Tosh is of a different nature. He seems to be completely unsure as to what he wants to do, and I have never had a patient this unsure who ever stuck with my program, which is very rigorous.

Mr. Tosh has already spoken to my colleague Dr. Wynder not once, but several times at great length regarding my work. Mr. Tosh was been in touch with our office many weeks ago, then never got back in touch with us.

We receive 25–30 calls every day from patients around the world requesting information on our program. I can only see 2–3 new patients a day at most, so we currently are turning down the majority of patients who want our treatment. This is unfortunate, but we are forced into a situation where we must choose our patients very carefully. When patients need to be convinced, we find it better to send them on to another treatment. While it may seem unfair, I simply do not have the resources to spend hours and hours trying to convince a patient to do the therapy.

I hope this helps.

Sincerely,
Nicholas Gonzalez, M.D.

27 September 1994

Dear Dr. Gonzalez

Thank you very much for your prompt reply. There seems to have been a misunderstanding regarding Mr. Gearin-Tosh. No one can be expected to make up their minds on any issue without specific information, particularly when life and death is at stake, and one has a rigorous academic training. It is this that has eluded Mr. Gearin-Tosh so far.

Dr. Wynder, with whom he has only spoken once, did not enlighten him as to the rationale and results of your therapy with multiple myeloma . . .

Mr. Gearin-Tosh is a very disciplined person, very stoical and courageous, and he would be capable of any rigorous regime, provided he can be given good reasons. At present he and I know nothing. Please reconsider and enlighten us. Surely you might have something in print at least? What about Kelley's book? Can we get that? Is he not your precursor?

Yours sincerely,
Dr. Carmen Wheatley

There is no reply.

I show these letters to Christian as we meet for lunch.

"Is Carmen Spanish?" asks Christian.

"You see her as a matador?" I reply.

"Well, we doctors know how to soft soap each other."

"I think Dr. Gonzalez is a brilliant man."

"He is also generous," says Christian. "He wants you to know that myeloma patients can do well."

"He probably thinks the calls that David Ambrose made to Wynder in fact came from me. That would explain the phrase in his letter that I spoke to Wynder 'several times at great length.' "

"And Dr. Gonzalez is very busy. Everyone forgets how busy doctors are. I certainly know."

"You have amazing energy."

"If only I did, Michael. What about the Gerson therapy?"

"Bad luck there too."

"How?"

"Gerson wrote a large book."

"Is that it?"

"Yes."

Christian takes my copy and flips through it.

"Very detailed," she says, "and look at these X-rays!"

"Rachel calls them nightmares."

"No. They are fascinating."

"Christian, I have read the text, and there is only one comment on myeloma."

I read it to her:

It may be added that leukemias and myelomas need greater doses of liver juice and vitamin B_{12} . . . their metabolisms are much "deeper" and more differently deranged than in other cancer types.

(*A Cancer Therapy,* p. 81)

And, regarding the vital liver juice, there is a reference in Appendix III:

On October 3, 1989, the Gerson Institute reached the conclusion that raw veal liver juice must be discontinued . . . this was based on multiple outbreaks of campylobacter gastroenteritis.

(*A Cancer Therapy,* p. 421)

"So I am deranged, more than in other cancers, and the remedy is deranged too."

"Michael, I think you are more pedantic than deranged."

"I must not whine."

"Really no," Christian giggles. "You are not a whiner."

"But how about this?"

I show her another book. It describes a visit to the Gerson clinic in Mexico:

The unmistakable powerful aroma of the Hippocrates soup hit me as I walked in. The world may turn somersaults, I thought with amusement, galaxies may rise and fall, but wherever Gerson patients foregather, the Hippocrates soup bubbles on.

(Beata Bishop, *A Time To Heal,* p. 299)

"Sounds like witches," says Christian. "Have you made this soup?"

"Not yet."

"Give me a report from the battlefront if you do. In the meantime, thank God for pasta."

We tuck into our lunch.

"Is Oxford term about to start?" asks Christian.

"Yes."

"What are you going to do?"

"I do not know. Can I do my job?"

"What do you think?"

"Pass."

"Give it a try. I know you are still anaemic, on the other hand I dislike you being alone, and you love the work. What about Rachel Trickett?"

"Very anxious."

"I thought 'so."

The book that mentions Hippocrates' soup is by Beata Bishop, who overcame cancer of the skin by the Gerson therapy.

Dr. Courteney Mayers tells me that Beata Bishop is to address a meeting in London. He is going: would I like to come? The subject of the talk is how to use meditation in cancer therapy.

You would not think from Beata Bishop's appearance and energy that she was a former cancer patient.

She demonstrates a technique in which the first part is

breathing and the second visualisation. But here the resemblance to my Chinese exercise stops. Instead of the Chinese elaboration the breathing in Beata Bishop's exercise is simple and practical: no breathing through the toes, let alone the bones of the skull. And her visualisations are sensitive and accessible, miles apart from the dramas of my borsch kitchen or my tunnels.

Do I change to Beata's exercises?

They are more simple.

But is it the very elaboration of the Chinese procedures that gives me a chance? Also, I now associate the Chinese exercise with escape. This is not strictly in focus: Dr. de Vries discovered the exercise while working at a country hospital in China. But the fact that his father survived Nazi labour camps even if he got cancer in them, the fact of Dr. H.'s escape from Vietnam, the fact that Dr. Gerson had to flee Europe because of the Nazis . . . all this forms a nexus of a kind. Not much of a kind, but there you are.

The Chinese exercise, too, is aimed specifically at the centre of the bones.

I shall stick with it.

9

OCTOBER WEEK 1

Oxford University is a confederation of forty Colleges, each of which is self-governing. Some colleges are ancient: University College, for example, may have been founded by King Alfred the Great (c. 847–99), and was certainly flourishing by the mid-thirteenth century. Corpus Christi College, my undergraduate college, was founded in 1517.

My own college, St. Catherine's, is modern. The foundation stone was laid by Her Majesty the Queen in 1960. St. Catherine's is slightly larger than many colleges. It consists of more than fifty Fellows or academics, of whom I am one. The Fellows form the Governing Body of the College and they appoint the Master, the administrative and academic head of the College.

We have just chosen a new Master.

Lord Plant was Professor of Political Philosophy at Southampton University. His books include a study of Hegel. He is also an active politician in the Labour Party.

When we interviewed him as a potential Master, he told us that as a young man he tried to become a monk. He started to train at an eminent institution and his spiritual life made progress. But he was defeated by two things. The first was the food. The second was the Abbot, who asked one day, "Do you think, Plant, you could learn to love me?"

Raymond Plant left, married and became an academic.

Lord Plant gives me a businesslike welcome, and walks without comment to his study. I know that he is within his rights to retire me. Someone has to do my job: I am Senior English Tutor, there are up to forty students, and there are the administrative and academic jobs that are a large part of the life of any Oxford don.

Lord Plant begins with the detachment of a philosopher. "I observe that there are two medical options. One option is to have chemotherapy at once. This is the advice of your first consultant. It is repeated, in essence, by the Harley Street consultant, by Professor Salmon in Arizona, by Dr. Tim Littlewood and Dr. Ray Powles. There is a different option, indeed a contrasting one: *If your friend touches chemotherapy, he's a goner.* These are the words of Professor Wynder. It seems to be the view—though here I make inferences—of Dr. de Vries, Dr. H. and Dr. Gerson.

"Is it the view of Dr. Carritt?" Lord Plant continues.

"She does not commit herself either way."

"And Dr. Wheatley?"

"She is a doctor of Donne and Spanish Literature."

"That makes a change."

He gives me a smile.

"How can these views be measured against each other?" he asks. "Option one, have chemotherapy, has the backing of all the cancer hospitals. On the other hand, you have Wynder, who is a big man, Dr. H. from Vietnam, Dr. de Vries, optimistic if mystical, and the late Dr. Gerson. No easy answers here. But it is four months since your diagnosis. The haemoglobin levels are up. Wynder and the rebels are rather my sort: I will recommend that the college support you."

Rachel springs a surprise. We must go together to St. Petersburg. For three weeks. The flat is full of brochures, maps and art books, which she has just bought.

"Michael darling, when you were there you cannot have had time to look at the Hermitage."

"Just an hour or so."

"I would love to see Rembrandt's *Prodigal Son.* They have Leonardos, Raphaels, Titians, stupendous Rubens landscapes. And Lely, Reynolds, Gainsborough and Morland. Stunning Lawrences. Let us go now, before it is cold."

"But I thought you did not like Russia."

"We are not going there to see Russian paintings. And will your friend, the Russian captain, be our bodyguard?"

(She had not wanted to meet Igor when he came, and up to now has described his visit as a freak.)

"But, Rachel, the term starts next week."

"You are not planning to teach?"

Her face says it all. Four months since diagnosis is survival for Lord Plant, but time running out for Rachel. Sweet love, she wants to give me a last treat.

OCTOBER WEEK 2

I see no point in concealing from my pupils that I have cancer. My finalists are passionate about their work, but they show grace and kindness: John Daniell, who plays rugby for his country, New Zealand; Antony Dunn, a poet; Atalanta Georgopoulos, also a poet; Simon Hollway, a brilliant and irreverent critic; and Rowan Joffé, who will take an outstanding first. My American students—I am a professor in the overseas department of Stanford—even organise a juice rota.

Oxford Colleges divide administrative jobs among their Fellows. Sod's law but I am in charge of the kitchens. As my food gets austere—even Gerson calls his regime "an unrelenting diet"—I am coaxing the kitchen into richer oxtail soups, grilled haggis, roast goose and fish cakes in the goose fat. My diet lapses in the face of a dish of scallops. Or a goats' cheese brie, ripe and running. And I sniff, even sip, when some wonderful claret is brought out for a special occasion. But in large part, I stick to boiled carrots, salad, porridge and fruit.

Joan Spencer comes to visit. She puts me in touch with a supplier who delivers organic vegetables each week. But there is an awkward moment.

"Claret?" accuses Joan, spying a bottle under the table.

It is beetroot juice.

OCTOBER WEEK 3

I am too busy with term to give thought to the material that Carmen sends.

She begs me, however, to take on board an article by Linus Pauling and Abram Hoffer. Published in 1993, it is an analysis of 134 patients "with advanced cancer": 101 were given vitamins, 33 not. Those with vitamins lived much longer. Pauling and Hoffer recommend that:

> all cancer patients begin the regimen as early in the course
> of the disease as possible, in addition to including fruits and
> vegetables in the diet:

Vitamin C	12 g
Vitamin B$_3$	1.5 to 3 g
Vitamin B$_6$	250 mg
Folic acid	5 to 10 mg
Other B vitamins	25 or 50 times RDAs
Vitamin E	800 I.U.
Beta carotene	25,000 I.U. to 50,000 I.U.
Selenium	0.2 to 0.5 mg
Zinc Citrate	50 mg

Sometimes calcium, magnesium, or a mineral tablet.

All or nearly of the nutrients are available without a prescription. We suggest checking the prices and not buying the high-priced preparations, even though claims of increased efficacy may be made for them . . .

Persons who have not developed cancer may find it wise to follow the regimen, perhaps with somewhat reduced amounts of the nutrients, to prevent or slow down the development of cancer and other diseases and to improve their general health and increase the length of their period of well-being and enjoyment of life.

(*Journal of Orthomolecular Medicine* 8, 1993, pp. 166–7)

OCTOBER WEEK 4

In their article Pauling and Hoffer go through the various types of cancer in their 134 patients. Nos. 258 and 270 are cases of myeloma.

No. 258 died a year after being first seen, but No. 270 was alive when the article was written.

Carmen, in her wonderful way, rings Canada and asks to speak to Dr. Hoffer.

He takes her call.

Yes, Patient No. 270 is still alive.

30 OCTOBER—5 NOVEMBER

Coffee enemas?

After all the fuss, I start. Echoing from my childhood came the Scots "no nonsense." Also I cannot find time to do the Chinese breathing exercise. I cannot relax enough. Perhaps the enemas will be a substitute.

I am also helped by Ronny Schwartz, who happens to phone as I am about to make my first experiment.

I tell her.

"Oh boy," Ronny says in a tone that I will not forget. I cannot flunk it now. The enema takes an hour. Dr. Gerson demands four enemas a day just as Dr. de Vries recommends three breathing exercises a day: how do patients find the time?

Off to London for acupuncture.

Dr. H. pulls up my shirt to put in the needles. He laughs.

"Skin yellow. Like canary."

"I am taking carrot juice."

"I have patient who die. She buy sacks of carrot every week."

"Cancer?"

"Yes. She buy sacks and sacks of carrots. Soon you look like a carrot."

Needles in. More laughter.

"But, Dr. H., your patient died?"

"She buy carrot twenty years. Yes, she die. Cancer. Die at ninety-four."

Dr. H. tells me that his father kept birds. As a boy in Saigon, they woke him every morning.

"Such a noise in the house. If there were any white canaries, they were fed carrots to make them orange."

NOVEMBER WEEK 1

I am seeing pupils, giving lectures and attending committees—the usual work of term.

I feel fine but there are days when I do not have time for breathing exercises and enemas.

Dr. Ray Powles of the Royal Marsden Hospital phones. When I met him in August, he asked me to ring if only to say how angry I was to have cancer. "And if you do not contact me, I will phone you."

We have a long chat.

"Would you consider trying a course of chemotherapy— just one—to see how you respond?" he asks.

I want to quote Wynder: *If your friend touches chemotherapy, he's a goner.* But I do not get round to it. Instead I invite him to a lecture by Peter Shaffer.

Dr. Powles accepts.

In his lecture, Peter Shaffer discusses the enlarging richness of Shakespeare:

> The wonder of Shakespeare is that he was intimidated by nothing. He avoided nothing. He had no time for the oblique in his handling of dramatic theme or of dominating emotion. Relentlessly, like the most fearless explorer which of course he was, he isolates in himself one major strand of

feeling with each major tragedy—pride, jealousy, infatua-
tion, ambition—seizes the end of it and pulls it clear out of
the psychic tangle within himself until it is all visible, iso-
lated in the brilliant magnifying light which only the artist
can switch on . . . Why have we so largely lost this *enlarging*
aspect of our work as playwrights?

Ray repeats Peter Shaffer's words to me at dinner:
Shakespeare was intimidated by nothing. Why am I intimidated
by cancer treatment? The treatment is developing all the
time. It can save my life.

An academic always returns a quotation. I cite the
famous lines on truth by John Donne:

> *. . . doubt wisely, in strange way*
> *To stand inquiring right, is not to stray;*
> *To sleep or run wrong is. On a huge hill,*
> *Cragged and steep, Truth stands, and he that will*
> *Reach her, about must, and about must go . . .*
>
> (Satire 3, lines 77–81)

Chemotherapy does not convince me: my position is
wise doubt.

"But you have doubted wisely," says Ray, "you have
obtained opinions throughout the world. And if you find a
better protocol of treatment, I will do it for you. But the
time has come for action. That is my professional advice.
Please take it seriously."

NOVEMBER WEEK 2

November keeps the warmth of September. It is an Indian summer. Roses flower. Lilies defy any touches of frost.

I read, teach and lecture as if cancer does not exist. I follow my diet, more or less. I drink juices. I have an enema some days. I am using them as a substitute for the breathing exercise, which I never have time for.

Rachel pines for a treat and we see an opera at Covent Garden.

NOVEMBER WEEK 3

Bad blood test. Haemoglobin results are as follows:

17.6.94	9.4
24.6.94	10.2
28.7.94	11.3
25.8.94	13.4
22.11.94	11.9

I am exhausted. Another test. Everything worse. Haemoglobin now 11.3, back to the level of July.

I am ill.

My colleagues take over the annual entrance exam.

Some weeks ago I found a helper who scrubs vegetables, makes juices, boils coffee and goes shopping.

He is now my lifeline.

I sleep in college so that I do not have to walk to Rachel's flat.

I am visited by Alan Bullock, the founding Master of my College and the historian of Hitler and Stalin.

Alan tells me that when he was Vice-Chancellor of Oxford University he presided over elections to Professorships. There would usually be seven electors, whatever the subject: some specialists, some outsiders, some with a senior academic position. There were lively debates. Elector X would attack the judgement of Elector Y, even Y himself or herself.

The exception was medicine. Medical electors would decide in advance who King Dog was, and when he or she barked the rest obeyed.

"Doctors are more like the army, Michael, than you can believe," Alan tells me. "There is no point in seeing more specialists. I believe you will only find a difference when you go to one of the great research doctors. Catch-22. They do not have patients. But we have an exception, here in Oxford. Our Regius Professor of Medicine is Sir David Weatherall, Fellow of the Royal Society. His Institute of Molecular Medicine is one of the great centres of research. David, however, is that rare combination, a researcher who also loves being a doctor. I once got him to tell me that a third of his time was spent on research, another third on administration—'totally wasted' as he put it—and a whole third on clinical work. Right through his career, he has looked after people as well as doing science. Let me write to him."

NOVEMBER WEEK 4

Another Fellow of the Royal Society visits me. Professor Sir James Gowans was for many years Secretary of the Medical Research Council in the UK and a Research Professor of the Royal Society. He has also been a Fellow of St. Catherine's College since 1961.

My colleagues have always spoken of him with awe. "He leaves for London at 4 a.m.," I was told as a young don, "and if you are ill he tells you to sort yourself out and waste doctors' time as little as possible." Years back there was a protracted crisis in college. I remember that James strode into a meeting, told us what to do in a few quiet words, and left almost at once. "Ruthless," said colleagues, but not to his face. What James advised, however, was the only way out of our crisis. But it took two months of hesitation, haggling and prevarication before a majority saw the point.

I get on with James, perhaps because we meet at plays and operas. He teases me for thinking that art conveys truths— this is a way of telling me to stop being solemn—but we will chat for weeks about a show.

His austerity of thought is offset by an extraordinarily open face and great courtesy. But he has unnerving powers of recall about a singer's note or the details of how a scene was acted.

James now looks me up and down as I lie in bed.

"Bad luck, Michael. But try to hang on. Old Professor —— had a leukaemia, but kept himself going. These diseases progress more slowly as you get older. How old are you?"

"Fifty-four."

"Professor —— was much older. My grandmother died in 1921 of diabetes. Do you know the significance of that medically?"

"No."

"If she lived one more year, they were starting to publish details of insulin treatment. I am glad that Alan Bullock is writing to David Weatherall."

"But will he see me?"

"I should think so. He is a saint when it comes to making time for people. Are you getting all the books you want?"

"Yes, but I do not feel like reading. I just sleep."

My helper wakes me for vegetable juices and light meals.

I fit in an enema every day. I should get up to two. And I start the breathing exercise again. It is feeble compared to what it was, and it takes a long time. But I get through it.

Ronny Schwartz is in California after an autumn in London.

She phones to see how I am, and I tell her the news.

"But you were fine when I came to Oxford in October. Let us get to work, Michael. If you do not mind, I will have a chat with Carmen."

From Scotland my mother worries that I am not in hospital. Rachel thinks the same. She tells my helper to have a break so that she can be alone with me.

"Michael, this helper is Carmen over again. He was a student of yours, he has no medical training. You are not in the jungle where you have to take any help that is going."

I tell Rachel that James Gowans came round.

She is astonished.

"Sir James Gowans saw you with that sack of dirty carrots in the corner, the juicer, the box of apples, enema bucket . . . What did he say?"

"Nothing about them."

"You have a world-class visitor in a room that looks like a slum. Talk about the saying that Oxford is high thinking but low living. You should be in a hospital."

"Rachel, can you imagine a hospital that tolerates vegetable juicers?"

"But what are you going to do next?"

"Get through today."

"You must have a plan."

"No. Have juices. Take the vitamins. Try breathing exercises. Get through tomorrow."

Is it unusual that the invalid has to spend time calming others?

Of course, it is wonderful that people care. But the energy of talking them down could be spent on getting well.

Anaemia is a medical enemy but a psychological friend. Anaemia prevents you doing almost all of what you want to do. This is maddening, except you do not have the energy to be angry. So you must select, and focus on the crucial.

A new way of shortening phone calls.

"Hi! Super of you to ring. May I explain that I am hitched to an enema bucket?"

A friend whom I do not have to calm is Drue Heinz. Rachel thinks that Drue's wealth—she is a benefactress to the University and many other causes—means that she must think in terms of up-to-the-minute, highly technological American medicine. In fact Drue both sifts the complex and values the simple.

She goes through the letters from my consultants.

"Why must they refer to what they do as 'proper' treatment? Is the rest improper? And who says?"

Drue invites me to stay when I come to see doctors in London.

"Bring your helper and stay in my guest flat as long as you need."

She also encourages me to persist with the juices and organic food.

"I cannot understand why people neglect diet. It stands to reason that you need the best nourishment if you are to mount a fight. Also the whole business keeps you busy."

It is a shrewd point. My days are spent in breathing exercises, juices and enemas. There is little time for melancholy: you are always assembling mental energy for the next routine.

Dr. Ray Powles writes to the college:

Dear Lord Plant,

As you know Michael Gearin-Tosh was diagnosed as having multiple myeloma in June. This is a difficult disease to bear and Michael does not lack a sense of what he is up against; he and Ronny Schwartz are in touch with a patient in the USA who has to live in a body brace.

I gather you have read that myeloma is incurable in Rees, Goodman and Bullimore, Cancer in Practice *(Oxford, 1993), but pilot work in the last few years is challenging this pessimistic outlook and although Michael was given a gloomy view of things at diagnosis he rightly refuses to accept it. He has had additional opinions at several hospitals and consultation with Professor Sydney Salmon in Arizona. Syd Salmon put Michael in touch with me because we have been a force in challenging the accepted inevitability of the perceived outcome of the disease.*

Our in-house data on patients like Michael with long follow-up makes me fairly certain I can offer Michael a good chance of significant survival if he accepts treatment. Obviously his age is a factor in this which reduces the death risk which always occurs and needs to be offset against the otherwise progressive nature of the disease.

Dr. Christian Carritt, who first sensed that Michael had a serious ailment, has urged caution. Professor Sir David Weather-

all will see Michael on the 20th January and obviously his opinion will be very important.

It is probable that Michael has had quite a long prodromal period before his disease was diagnosed, probably with associated anaemia and a reduction in energy, which will have impaired his health and output perhaps for several years. The longest instance I have known of myeloma being prodromal is greater than ten years.

Michael has put himself under a rigorous discipline in fighting the disease. Whatever we decide to do I feel strongly the College and University should grant him sick leave for the January/February Term. He is not strong enough to be in post at present, although he insisted on working last term in order to welcome his new colleague, Dr. White, and while Dr. Wordsworth took sabbatical leave. His medical results deteriorated significantly during November. Michael needs rest and help if he is to fight this disease, not least because he has spirit and is so brave.

The support of his friends is quite astonishing. I trust that College and the University will accede to my recommendations, and that you will be good enough to forward my letter to relevant authorities.

> *Your sincerely,*
> *Dr. R. L. Powles MD BSc FRCP FRCPath*
> *Head & Physician in Charge,*
> *Leukaemia and Myeloma Units.*

I need quiet.

Why not go to Scotland? I am not so ill that I cannot travel in a sleeper. Maria Whelan offers to come with me.

I shall be able to breathe mountain air.

I tell Benjamin Ross that I am going.

"But I will come too, Michael. Can I bring James?"

James Marsh was also my pupil at Oxford some ten or so

years ago. He now works for the BBC as a director of documentaries. He is between schedules and he can take a week off.

Oxford is often criticised for being a university for the elite. All of us who work there have examples of the opposite.

James Marsh came for our entrance interviews while living in a squat in South London. He was eighteen, working-class and estranged from his father; his mother was dead.

It is characteristic of him that he did not mention his circumstances at the time.

When James was in the middle of his degree course I came back to Oxford one August and found him working in the kitchen for conferences. Not the worst of jobs, but much more pleasant in winter than in a humid Oxford summer.

Students benefit from a gap year before they start their studies.

Most students travel. Some work in charities in Nepal or Morocco, others backpack in Australia or South America. If students come from poor families, I put them in touch with sources of help. James Marsh's reticence at the entrance interviews meant that we did not know that the gap year would cause him problems.

He went to Israel and worked on a kibbutz. His money and clothes were stolen. He moved to Tel Aviv and washed dishes, living in a work hostel. But another worker assaulted him. He then lived on the beach. Once he was arrested and spent three days in jail.

"The jail was part of a tourist police station, so it could have been worse," he told me.

In the end he washed enough dishes to pay for a flight home.

As I write, James Marsh lives in New York and achieves distinctions in his career as a maker of documentary films. His *Wisconsin Death Trip* (1999) is premiered at the Venice Film Festival and wins a FIPRESCI award at the San Sebastian Festival. It is shown with acclaim in the commercial cinema in the United States, and is screened in the UK by BBC2.

10

My diary is incomplete for the days in Scotland and I rely on the memories of Benjamin and James.

Both think the journey to Scotland was a bad idea and exhausted me.

"One night we thought you might be dying," says Benjamin. "You spent hours violently coughing up white foam. But you also insisted on your routines. You had enemas, and Maria and James made you juices. But I was no help. Kate's death had totally spun my head and James was babysitting me. God knows how we coped. I felt at home with you because you and I were both on the edge."

"I was struck by the pace," remembers James. "You were very ill and various doctors rang up, but you were not prepared to trust anyone's judgement. My hope was that you would be able to keep on looking things in the eye and being practical. You insisted on going for very short walks most days, just into the garden. The weather was foul. You also forced yourself to bake bread. The therapy said to have bread with no salt, and we could not buy any."

"Maria was amazing," says Benjamin, "and James had just met Anna Mehta [to whom he is now married]. A third pillar of sanity was Jimmy Hewitson, who always managed to make us think that normal life was somehow continuing. A crisis came for us, but it passed."

Back to London. Drue Heinz passes a high test of friendship: who else would let Mayfair be invaded by coffee enemas? My helper comes to stay and joins me in Drue's guest flat.

I consult doctors. "Rest," says Dr. H. "Do only what you can," prescribes Christian.

Drue's flat is quiet and my days are a routine of breathing exercises, juices, enemas, short walks and sleep.

Drue coaxes me out now and then. She wants me to see that I can still be a part of life, although she is too skilful to put this into words. She finds a Lebanese restaurant that can approximate to my diet. We go to a screening in Soho with Benjamin. Friends unobtrusively join her in stopping me from being cut off, Olga Polizzi, Tessa Keswick, Romilly McAlpine, Aru, Rufus and Michael Codron: did they form a rota? Benjamin and James come round when they can.

My plan is to join Rachel for Christmas in Oxford. She has friends to stay as usual, and our flat will be very festive. But I am spitting up foam again, and the weather is bitter.

Drue goes away for Christmas, and my helper must join his family.

I persuade Rachel that it is best for me to stay at Drue's. She worries that I will be alone, but Shawais, my Kurdish friend, finds a refugee from Albania who offers to come and make a couple of juices each day.

When I go to pay the Albanian on his first visit he refuses the money.

"You need it more than I do."

And he does not come again.

•   •   •

Benjamin sits with me on Boxing Day, and we chat about the Albanian.

Did I seem too feeble?

Might my death bring him bad luck?

Anyway we manage to cope. Benjamin makes juices. Christian cooks me supper one evening, and Tessa and Henry Keswick ask me for New Year.

Drue comes back and insists on a party. There are only two of us, but we celebrate.

We get into a conversation about Impressionist painters. We both love Manet and think water lily Monet is overrated.

"Did you know," asks Drue, "that Manet painted the *Bar at the Folies Bergères* when he was dying?"

"No."

Drue has the catalogue of the great 1983 Manet exhibition that she saw in New York and I had seen in Paris. We read that Manet was not yet fifty when he did the painting and that he died the following year. In *Bar at the Folies Bergères* a barmaid stands and faces us. In a mirror behind her—the first time Manet used a mirror, says the catalogue—customers relax at their tables and drink beneath the chandeliers. The barmaid is young and beautiful but with red hands and, as the catalogue puts it, "mélancolie du regard absent." By a trick of perspective, we also see in the mirror the man she is talking to. Perhaps he is trying to pick her up. He is puffy, unwell and not attractive.

"But how Manet loves life and people," says Drue, "and how he wants to celebrate them until the end."

The UK closes down for a long time between Christmas and the end of the New Year holiday. The days are damp and dark, but though I am often alone in the flat things happen.

The breathing exercises are easier.

At times in the past I have had to lie for an hour before I was relaxed enough to start. Now I am so exhausted that five minutes is enough. And I manage two sessions every day, even the three that Dr. de Vries recommends. I need to straighten my skeleton as I go through each part. I have a struggle with my right shoulder, which tends to be out of alignment.

In the visualisation part of the exercise, the borsch kitchen and Russian troops disappear. Without any scene-setting, I travel down tunnels and hunt cancer cells. The tunnels are not dark or claustrophobic. And I am unaware how I travel: I could be on skis or on a mechanical walkway. The action is wholly concentrated on finding enemy cells and destroying them.

Russia leaves the visualisations, but joins the enemas. I develop a need to read about Russia so that I can relax enough to start the enemas. And I continue reading afterwards as I sit on the loo. If I try to read anything else, my mind refuses.

There are memoirs of the Kutuzov period in Drue's library. One is by Cornélie de Wassenaer, a Dutch lady who went to St. Petersburg at the end of the reign of Alexander I, the Czar of Kutusov. How can I complain about a dark London Christmas when Cornélie writes that she saw no sun for fifteen days?

Cornélie was an heiress and she was entertained at court. Luxury, however, did not protect her but generated its own bad weather:

> It was the Grand Duke Michael's birthday and a ball was given in his honour in the White Hall, so called because it is white stucco with white marble columns which were hung with wreaths of lighted candles, not perhaps very prettily

arranged but emphasizing the brilliance of the room by their mere numbers. What is more, the marble sweated and the heat transformed this damp into a sort of mist that filled the card-room.

(Cornélie de Wassenaer, *A Visit to St. Petersburg,* p. 81)

Cornélie describes other details of court life:

I could not help staring with amazement at the thin waists of the officers of the Empress's regiment who stood against a window and looked so transparent that you could have cut them in half like wasps.

All Russian officers are so terribly tight-laced that they can hardly sit down. Apart from the shell jacket and the belt which had to be pulled tight by two men, so I was told by an officer himself, they wear skin-tight breeches down to their high boots, which makes it impossible for them to bend their knees.

Even the royal males were corseted: "The Imperial family is no exception." Also young men:

From early youth the cadets are laced like this in the various schools, which makes their chests stick out as though they were stuffed.

This unnatural state of things makes them die before their time and it is very rare for a Russian soldier to finish his period of service, supposed to last twenty-five years irrespective of the age at which he enrolled.

(*A Visit to St. Petersburg,* p. 45)

Does she exaggerate? Probably. But her images are memorable: a political elite that does not allow itself to breathe, let alone anyone else; gross luxury generating a damp in which you would not breathe freely even if you could.

Cornélie met the cruelty of Russia as soon as she crossed the border:

> I cannot describe how melancholy I felt the first time I saw a peasant patiently accept a blow from a postmaster's switch without seeming to mind any more than an ordinary man would mind a word of reproach. His heavy sheepskin was bound to lessen the force of the blow but it did not seem any less of an outrage to me.
>
> (*A Visit to St. Petersburg,* p. 36)

I am to immerse myself in Russia for many months. It becomes a compulsive need. Why? Is it escapism? Cancer doctors have a habit of accusing patients of escapism: I seem to get it regularly.

But put my reading about Russia in context.

If you have a cancer that is attacking your skeleton, is there escapism in the Chinese breathing exercise? You really get to know each bone: you breathe up and down it, up seven times, down seven times, and when you cross over you breathe a further seven times each way. Twenty-eight times per bone per session. And I was doing two or three sessions each day.

Or enemas. Two pints of coffee up your colon is a distinct reminder that you are not well. Three times a day. Not to mention vegetable juices and a daily injection.

Thus a large part of my day is spent on cancer. Every day.

How are you to spend the rest?

Letting your fears surface? Panic? Weighing the odds of what you do against the fact that orthodox doctors consider you "crazy"?

Or do you spend the spare hours living somewhere else in imagination?

The Marchioness of Londonderry, an English battleaxe, visited Russia in the 1830s, during the reign of another Czar whom I dislike, Nicholas I. She wrote a journal which is among Drue's books and, like Cornélie, she met officers:

> I never saw education so carefully attended to nor so much observance of duty and respect to decorum. The good of all this system is seen in the conduct of the young people . . . discipline is early introduced among the boys and submission, respect and obedience impressed. The young men are all brought up to serve whether in the military or civil or diplomatic service, and this is universal however high the rank or large the fortune. The greater part are in the army. No officer is ever seen out of uniform. I asked Monsieur Novosiltzov, aide de camp of the Governor of Moscow, to walk with me in the bazaar of Moscow if he could put on plain clothes. "Moi! Madame, je suis né en uniforme, je suis venu au monde comme cela" was his reply.
> (*Russian Journal of Lady Londonderry 1836–7*, pp. 72–3)

Birth in corsets.
And, as ever, there was the climate:

> The cold had been daily increasing and now had arrived at nearly thirty degrees below zero. This is not to be imagined but is fearful when felt. Light furs feel like cold linen. The eyelashes are painful, the breath freezes, the windows become opaque, and a sickening feel pervades the whole frame as of a knife cutting to one's marrow.
> (*Russian Journal*, pp. 107–8)

Igor was unable to breathe good air in a Russian *summer.* As he told me, "The collective farm was disgusting. My God, you cannot imagine. Thirty kilometres from anywhere. Road too muddy for use five months. There was no river. Hot wind all summer. How could we breathe? By making a dark room with newspapers over the window . . . All we dreamed of was getting away."

My trap is cancer. No escape, even to a mild climate: Professor Salmon and Dr. Powles have ruled out air travel. The Czarist officers, in my case, come from hospitals that administer chemotherapy to prolong life but by a process of pain and nausea. It is easy to identify: Cornélie wrote of the same peasants who were whipped by the postmaster:

> I heard them singing a melancholy song. At the same time they are always shouting like madmen and this seems to act as a great stimulus both to them and to their horses.
>
> (*A Visit to St. Petersburg,* p. 36)

I start to shout in my visualisation tunnels. But I have a sneaking regard for the grand Russian ladies. Lady Londonderry could not "conceive how the women bear the cold":

> It is very true, one instant suffices to jump into a carriage. In full *toilette* these Russian ladies rush from a heat of twenty five degrees to a cold of twenty five below zero making a transition of fifty degrees in a moment.
>
> (*Russian Journal,* p. 108)

Sounds like tempering metal.
Tough blades.

JANUARY

No escape to warmth?

Ronny Schwartz rings.

She has a guest house on the beach in California: why do I not come out, she will fly me there, and she will buy a juicer so that I can continue with the Gerson therapy.

There is also a famous cancer hospital in La Jolla.

"You always love your American students," adds Ronny. "Come to the terrain."

Dr. Powles says that although he had advised against air travel, the benefits outweigh the risk.

I have never been to California and I start to dream of sun, beaches and quiet seas.

It is time for my appointment with Sir David Weatherall. I go to the Institute of Molecular Medicine, which is next to the John Radcliffe Hospital in Oxford. Sir David comes personally to reception and takes me to his study. In time I notice that no phones ring and no secretary comes in. All my medical records are on his desk, but Sir David asks me to state the case as I see it.

I go through my history.

Sir David does not say a word.

"Chemotherapy at once" was the advice of my first consultant, also from Harley Street. But there was "Touch chemotherapy and you are a goner" from Professor Wynder. Then chemotherapy was recommended by Professor Salmon in Arizona, Dr. Littlewood and Dr. Powles.

"I hope I have not been obstreperous in resisting this advice," I say.

"Obstreperous is too mild a word for you, Mr. Gearin-Tosh. But go on."

His face is still, but his eyes are laughing.

I continue with Dr. Gonzalez, Dr. de Vries, Dr. H. and Professor Sherman, the Columbia professor who suggested to Carmen that I might delay. I tell Sir David what I do. I go to Dr. H. for acupuncture and I follow the Gerson therapy: strict diet, vegetable juices, enemas, injections of liver juice and vitamin B_{12}. I also do Chinese bone breathing exercises. With visualisations.

I finish and there is silence.

"Do you think I am mad to try what I am doing?" I ask.

Sir David Weatherall is a man who thinks for as long as he wishes before he speaks.

A minute or two pass.

"What you must understand, Mr. Gearin-Tosh, is that we know so little about how the body works."

I am astonished.

Sir David repeats his remark.

"We know so little about how the body works."

Nine short words.

Blood rushes through my head. I could be floating in air.

Suddenly, Sir David starts to speak without a break.

No taciturnity.

He is talking me down.

Do I, he asks, have details of Wynder's career? It seems that Wynder practised what we might call orthodox cancer treatment for most of his life, but then he changed.

"Of course when people work at something every day, they have to believe in it: did you say that Wynder's last phase involved work on cancer statistics?"

Sir David is not taking sides: he puts two perspectives in balance with each other.

Carmen wanted me to ask Sir David about the use of interferons as a mild alternative to chemotherapy.

"I do not call that mild," says Sir David, and he takes me through an abstract of an article on interferon by Professor Sherman: "Toxicities include mild to moderate maculopapular rash . . . fevers to 104 degrees, malaise and hypotension . . ."

"*Fevers to 104 degrees:* I do not think anyone would wish to get more hot. May I put it this way? You have a swine of a disease. It is vital that you take care of yourself. Do not get tired. Do not get cold. Do not get wet. The University will support you in what you are doing, and if you need help do not hesitate for a second to ask. I am only a phone call away."

Sir David writes to Dr. Powles at the Royal Marsden Hospital:

> *University of Oxford*
> *Professor Sir David Weatherall FRS*
> *Regius Professor of Medicine.*
> *Jan 30*
>
> *Dear Ray,*
> *I have had two sessions with Michael Gearin-Tosh now, and we have come to some kind of compromise over his treatment.*
> *As you know he was very loath to undergo chemotherapy of any kind for the immediate future. He would, however, be willing to start treatment should his disease deteriorate. We agree, therefore, that the best approach would be for him to have a further biochemical profile carried out in London by your good self before he goes to California. Assuming there has been no major change he would take his various biochemical data with him to the States and be followed there with a further screen in*

a month or two. I gather that the lady who is organizing his stay in La Jolla has already made contact with Dr. Brouillard at the Scripps Clinic. He will then return for further studies at the Marsden when he comes back from the States.

He has agreed that if there is any change in the course of his illness, either clinical or if there is evidence of expansion of the tumour mass suggested by a change in the level of his paraprotein or anything else, he will be willing to undergo treatment.

I have warned him of the importance of maintaining contact with only a limited number of doctors in the future and strongly advised him that monitoring and treatment really should be carried out in one centre and that should be the Marsden with yourself. I am very happy to act as a kind of pastoral supporter here but if there is any serious treatment to be carried through, it should be at your end.

I am giving Michael a copy of this letter and he has copies of all your biochemical data so he will have plenty of material for his physicians in the States.

All best wishes,

Yours sincerely,
D. J. Weatherall

We know so little about how the body works: I know by instinct that this is a turning point, but not why. For some days my mind insists on being blank, and rejects everything, including the visualisation exercise. My mind will not allow me to do it. This is what happened after Dr. H. told me about his escape.

The word "perhaps" echoes about. Where from? Is it the *perhaps* that I picked up from Dr. Barlogie's remark *when perhaps the immune system can cope*. An undermining *perhaps* in that context, I had thought, an admission of doubt by Barlogie, but wise doubt, a limit to certainty about the success of his procedures. Perhaps uncertainty is centre stage for all doctors. Why have I been so slow to see this?

Yet only Sir David puts the point to me as a patient.

He is a contrast to the others. The knowingness and bullying of my first consultant, the cricket player's bonhomie of Harley Street, Professor Salmon reacting as if his hearing aid needed adjustment . . . are these the habits people pick up when they have to cope with a situation about which they know little but cannot say so?

Not that any of the three consultants were ill intentioned. Imagine the career prospects of a consultant who, on the usual pyramid of secretaries, nurses, students, white hospital buildings and long corridors, smiles at a patient with, "I know so little about what is wrong with you. Or, indeed, what is right."

Sir David Weatherall has a fellow spirit in Christian Carritt. Not that Christian expresses things in his way. But by giving me time to think for myself, she has prepared the ground for Sir David.

"Weatherall felt he could be straightforward with you," says James Gowans. "It is a clinician's skill, and a very difficult one, to sense what can be said to a patient. Although David is a great scientist, he is also a superb doctor. A rare combination."

David Weatherall also asks a former pupil of his, Dr. Neil Maclennan, to be my GP.

When I go to Dr. Maclennan's practice in Beaumont Street, Oxford, I am greeted by its former head, Dr. Godfrey Fowler, who is now the Reader in Clinical Medicine in the University.

"The University set up a Department of General Practice in the 1970s," he tells me, "and I have established a number of courses in so-called complementary therapies."

As we chat, Dr. Fowler says that in an ideal world anthropology should be a part of medical education, as it is in Norway. He certainly considers that how a patient experiences medicine is a neglected aspect of study. Dr. Fowler also tells me that, as a doctor, he has conducted over a quarter of a million consultations in the course of his life. He regards medicine as full of uncertainties and that sharing these uncertainties with a patient is an important aspect of developing the patient's trust.

FEBRUARY

Russians calculate Christmas and Easter by "the Old Calendar." Christmas Day is 7 January, and a card comes from Igor with this letter:

My dear friend!

HOW ARE YOU? I'm worriing about you and I wish you all the best!

Michael! I'm in the hospital now. I'm here for 2 or 3 weeks only. I have problems with my nose. This hospital is near Moscow (Podolsk), 45' from Moscow.

One telephone for 9 floors, 8 or 9 people in one room, terrible foods. I forget when I was eating fruit.

But do not worry. My doctor'll give me 3 days off after of the cure. I'm glad.

Sometimes I seem I receive the letter from you where you'll write: "Igor, my doctor told me my diagnosis is mistake. I'm fine."

I wish you it.
Write me. Take care.

                    Igor.

I tell Rachel about Ronny Schwartz's offer to fly me to California. Rachel is upset but she will not tell me why. I suspect that she has turned the textbook on cancer into an Old Testament prophecy: "Multiple myeloma is incurable. The median survival time from clinical confirmation to death is under a year in untreated patients." My illness since November confirms everything. She will not quite put it into words, but her thought is: why do I want to die in California?

I confer with Carmen, and she gallantly offers to phone Rachel.

They chat for half an hour about the advantage of California sun, its effect on the bones, the fact that La Jolla is a quiet resort and has a famous cancer hospital.

"The surprise," Rachel growls, "is that Michael's life is so mouvementé."

How can I calm Rachel? She likes Ronny—"Bryn Mawr mind, always questioning"—but it makes no difference. Will it help if I bring Rachel and Christian together?

Rachel always enjoys seeing John Bayley, so I find an evening when he will be in St. Catherine's and I invite Christian as well. Rachel is on form with John, but talks to Christian for no more than a minute.

Next day at breakfast, and from behind *The Times*, Rachel says, "A very beautiful woman, your friend Carritt."

"I am glad you liked her."

"It is not a question of liking. You are always too influenced by appearance."

I keep quiet.

"The point about Carritt is that she is sound."

"I am pleased you think so."

"It is not what I think. I do not have imaginary competencies, like Carmen."

Coffee is stirred.

The quality of *The Times* has gone down, I am told. Further. Why print attacks on the Book of Common Prayer? As for these trashy columnists . . .

"Go and scrub your carrots. Dame Janet knew that Carritt was sound."

The mafia of lady dons.

Christian Carritt was an undergraduate at Somerville College, Oxford, when Dame Janet Vaughan was Principal. Dame Janet died a year ago but Rachel has made enquiries and elicited this piece of information, which possibly dates back forty years.

Life may do to you what it will, but how you were at twenty for a great lady is how you are at sixty.

I knew Janet Vaughan a little, and I thought it a great privilege. She was a research doctor and her particular interest was blood and marrow. By a quirk of fate she spent the last weeks of the Second World War as leader of a small team investigating how to treat starvation in liberated Europe. This took her to Belsen.

When she died in 1993 Somerville College published a letter that she wrote to a friend from the camp:

12v45

My dear Molly

   I am here—trying to do science in hell—A stench of faeces & rags, rubbish heaps & dead bodies hangs heavy in the air—Dead bodies of men, women & children lie about in heaps along the road side & among the fine trees—In the huts the dead & the living lie in heaps together—from such heaps my patients come—Poles & Russians, French & Dutch, Czechs & Hungarians, men & women, children & pregnant women & infants—There is Typhus & dysentery, diphtheria & scarlet fever & over all & everything there is human excreta—endlessly & unceasingly—I give a transfusion with one hand & wave a bedpan with the other. I talk Science to peripatetic Americans—Human skeletons scratch in rubbish heaps outside my window for rags to wear—Men & Women walk about in nakedness crying for bread—some are mere skin & white with famine oedema—When they come in to my special ward they shriek "Nicht Crematorium, nicht crematorium" especially the young men—they shiver away in terror when I come near—they cannot believe or understand kindliness—Syringes before meant injections of benzene the better for burning—alive—

At night a cart comes round in the sunset to collect the nameless dead—we bury them 5000 at a grave—Many of them in the past intellectuals of great charm—

War is perhaps understandable—it is killing—but this one will never understand . . .

I shall be back in ten days . . . here we have lost all sense of time—our realities are so different . . . yet to have had even a share in it has been a great though terrible experience—it could never be realised in its full horror unless one had seen & heard & smelt it.

Yours ever,
Janet Vaughan

The young Janet got into Oxford as a student only at the fourth attempt. She was dyslexic, which may have held her back. When she was a student one of her contemporaries said that it was impossible to invite her to a party because she was always in tweeds.

She acted, wrote poetry and she was awarded a first in Physiology in 1922.

When Janet Vaughan was twenty-six, Virginia Woolf, who was a cousin of her father, described her as "good, dull Janet Vaughan." Some dullness . . . (It may be noted that Virginia Woolf changed her opinion, fractionally, two years later. She wrote in her diary for 1928 that Janet Vaughan "is an attractive woman; competent, disinterested, taking blood tests all day to solve some abstract problem.")

I have not associated Christian with Janet Vaughan. But I start to see Christian's spirit in what has been written about Dame Janet.

In a memorial address, Barbara Harvey, a former colleague, gave this memory:

> She was accessible and exhilarating. Of course, we noticed that she was partial, but I suppose that we learnt to take this in our stride. It was exhilarating to have a Principal who made no secret of her own views, however controversial. Although we half smiled, as I think she did too, at her expressed conviction that a Somervillian put down anywhere in the world, in any situation, whatever the odds, would know how to cope, many of us left Oxford wondering whether there might not, after all, be something in the idea . . . Few heads of houses can have exerted more influence over their societies than she did over hers.

Philippa Foot, the philosopher and Fellow of Somerville, has written that:

Janet's generosity was legendary and no task was too menial for her if it needed to be done. When there was a flu epidemic she was the first to carry trays. To be sure she had occasionally bitten one's head off, but that was part of the price one paid for the immense privilege and the excitement of working with her.

On one occasion, the fiancé of a student was invited by Dame Janet to stay in her own house.

When he came down on Sunday, he found the great lady in her dressing gown busily frying him a plateful of sausages. A grand gesture of welcome resulted in the sausages flying out of the pan, but they collected them up, brushed them down and ate them happily.

MARCH

I have lunch with Christian before leaving for California.

"Did Janet Vaughan teach you?"

"No," says Christian, "she was my Principal."

"Who was your tutor?"

"Anyone who could face it. In my last year they all refused."

"Seriously?"

"I never wanted to do Medicine. The first I knew about it was when I was still at school. The House Mistress had me in. 'So nice, Christian, to have someone who is definite about a career.' Do you know, my mother had written to the House Mistress and told her that I was trying for Medicine at Oxford?"

"Just like that?"

"Yes."

"And you were not interested in Medicine?"

"No. Never crossed my mind to study it."

"Amazing."

"My dear, I nearly passed out. I went and sat on the loo for two hours. At least if I get into Oxford, I thought, I can be together with my brother, who was there. I adored him more than anything in the world."

"Was your mother very perceptive? Her intuitions . . ."

"It was all very odd: she was, in a way, a doctor manqué herself. What are you smiling at?"

"Just a thought."

"Yes?"

"It was Chekhov's mother who told him to be a doctor."

"Really?"

"She just wrote and put it to him. We have the letter. So long live mothers' instincts for making doctors!"

"But I never studied. I was always falling in love. The tutors wrote ghastly reports about me. 'But I do not worry about you,' Janet Vaughan would say, 'it is those who are bored with life, I cannot stand. Fail your exams, you will sit them again.' "

"Did she influence you?"

"Janet Vaughan sent me to University College Hospital, which is where I started to like Medicine. I have a talent for patients. It is the right job for me, I have no doubt about that. But I should have studied: I would like to be more knowledgeable. Anyway, have you been to California before?"

"No. I hope I am strong enough to get there."

"Are you going alone?"

"A pupil is coming. I need help with the carrots."

"I suppose, if one is not up to it, the juice never gets made."

"Nor the enemas."

"How many a day?"

"Supposed to be four. I do not get beyond two."

"Well done for that."

"Christian, I remember Janet Vaughan. I first met her with Rosemary Woolf and then from time to time with Rachel. She was down to earth but also like air on a mountain."

"You could not meet anyone less claustrophobic. A thing I hate about modern doctors is that they will not examine properly. Take cancer of the bowel. They will not examine shit."

"I bet Dame Janet would."

"Of course. Or take counselling. It is everywhere now. But what sick people really need is humanity and kindness."

"Chekhov made a wonderful remark: 'the nearer a person is to truth, the more intelligent and simple they are.' Is that not Janet Vaughan?"

Somehow we get on to Dame Janet's sausages, flung about, "brushed down" and eaten.

"I cannot take hygiene either," says Christian.

Chekhov also surfaces in my last evening with Rachel.

"Michael, was Chekhov a serious doctor?"

"He practised all his life."

"It is very unusual to be a great dramatist and have another career, and certainly one not connected with the theatre."

"But it is a tradition in Russia for doctors to be literary. Russians even have a joke that you must not think that because you practise medicine you can manage prose."

"Would not raise a laugh here."

"No."

"Do we know what Chekhov thought about cancer?"

"He believed you should never separate mind and body in serious illness."

"But did he have cancer patients?"

"Yes, many. And there is a wonderful letter."

"Will you read it to me?"

I get my copy of Chekhov's *Letters*. Rachel takes it and looks at the photo of Chekhov.

"Michael, it is a very patient face."

"And a patient's face."

"He died of tuberculosis?"

"Yes. At forty-four."

"You love him, don't you?"

"Yes."

"But he is rough on doctors in the plays."

"Rachel, you are off again."

"No. Not beyond the evidence. There is the drunk doctor in *Three Sisters* and a matinee idol doctor in *Vanya* who forgets his patients so as to hang about hoping for the Professor's wife."

"There is an even worse doctor."

"Who?"

"Dr. Lvov in *Ivanov*. Chekhov wrote that he was 'the model of an honest, straightforward, hot-headed but narrow-minded and limited man.' "

"Anything else?"

"Yes. 'He's walking ideology. He looks at every phenomenon and person through a narrow frame . . .' "

"Spot on."

"But, Rachel, there are people like that in any profession."

"Darling, you are very obstinate in favour of doctors."

"Rachel, you love some doctors."

"Do I?"

"Janet Vaughan."

This throws Rachel.

Yes, she had the highest regard for Dame Janet, and she reveres her memory.

"I suppose I have always thought of her as head of an Oxford college, as my colleague, not as a doctor. And though Janet loved to gossip, she was totally discreet about patients. But you are right. And you have me on two scores, since she also liked Russia. She went behind the Iron Curtain and I remember how she entertained Akhmatova in Oxford. But it is beyond me, Michael, why you all like Russia. You do agree that they have had a terrible history? Anyway, what about this Chekhov letter on cancer? Is it distressing?"

"Sort of. It is tough."

"Pass. Do not read it. Pour me a malt instead."

Benjamin phones to say that the studio wants him in Los Angeles while I will be in California. He schedules time to come and stay with me for a week.

Ronny Schwartz has a last-minute surprise.

"Michael, why do you not ask the Russian captain to come to California? It is good for you to have company. I would send him a ticket."

Igor cannot believe his luck.

He rings me back next day.

"The commander is astonished. He grants me leave."

Maria Whelan, my pupil, drives with me to Gatwick. We change at Dallas and step out into the warmth of San Diego, where Ronny meets us.

An incredulous Igor flies in two days later.

I have to frog-march him through the car park at San Diego airport.

"Is he exhausted after the journey?" asks Ronny.

Only now as I write, does Igor explain. His mother had seen Soviet films in which America is the land of gangsters. Vehicles are always being sabotaged with bombs. She told Igor not to walk close to a car.

11

I stop my account at the end of twelve months (March 1994 to April 1995). I have delayed writing for seven years since medicine has a saying that if the patient is alive after five years the disease has gone away.

I have added elements to my therapies and much has changed in Chekhov's "psycho-organic" sense. But that is another story.

Year by year, I have more energy. But my haemoglobin remains depressed—Carmen calls me "sub-anaemic"—and my immune system is disordered.

Another problem is my bones. They were first tested in California and they were found to be much too thin.

"For God's sake, do not take up parachuting," said Ray Powles.

There is a gruesome patient in Solzhenitsyn's *Cancer Ward* who welcomes newcomers with: "Even if they *do* let you go home, you'll be back here pretty quick. The Crab [cancer means crab] loves people. Once he's grabbed you with his pincers, he won't let you go till you croak" (Part I, chapter 2).

I am not so rash as to think I have escaped.

•   •   •

I continue to see all of the people in my book and I am in touch with Igor. But Rachel is no longer here.

There is a huge void in my life.

John Bayley wrote this obituary when she died in June 1999:

> Rachel Trickett, who has died aged 78, was the daughter of a Wigan postman. She became Principal of St. Hugh's College, Oxford from 1973 to 1991. She often spoke of her happy childhood, and of her father's love for books. He usually had a sample of his current reading in his post-bag, and would recommend it or not, as the case might be, to the friends and neighbours to whom he was delivering the mail. He and his daughter were greatly attached and she caught his reading habit at a very early age. This relationship forms the background of her first work of fiction, *The Return Home* (1952), a moving novel of subtlety and refinement which is a masterpiece and a highly original one.
>
> Always very much a Lancashire lass in her speech, her robust manner and her fearless independence of thought . . . She became a highly successful if sometimes controversial Principal of St. Hugh's College. She was always on the side of gaiety and unusualness.
>
> (*The Guardian*, 30 June 1999)

from Sir David Weatherall FRS
University of Oxford

Living Proof *does underline the extraordinary chasm between the world of complementary medicine and conventional western medical practice. Human beings are unbelievably complex organisms about which we understand very little. I suspect that the fruits of the genome project will take years to unravel and it will be even longer before we understand how the human brain works and how it can influence organic disease elsewhere in the body. Though I do believe passionately in scientific medicine, I have not got to the stage of being so blinkered that I cannot believe that at least some aspects of the more complementary approach to medicine may have a lot to offer. I think they could be put to scientific test, and should be, but whether this will happen is far from clear. But of one thing I am sure; regardless of what a patient is suffering from, their reaction to their situation, and their state of mind, is of critical importance and to ignore it in the face of high technology and medical practice is to court disaster.*

You have done wonderfully well and the message of Living Proof *is very far reaching. It should certainly make all of us in conventional medicine feel a little uncomfortable and teach us an enormous amount about the stresses and strains of living under the cloud of serious disease. You do a great service to us all.*

from Professor Robert A. Kyle (i)
Mayo Clinic, Rochester, Minnesota, USA

Whether or not one agrees with the therapeutic modalities, Living Proof *is worthwhile reading for all physicians. Michael Gearin-Tosh is a wonderful writer. The reader feels that he is experiencing some of the same things that the patient is undergoing. All physicians should read it in order to obtain a better understanding of the effect their conversation, advice and interest has upon the patient.*

The comments concerning rudeness are really true and are well stated.

Dr. Carritt's comments about statistics are important. I always emphasise to patients that statistics are of little or no value to them as an individual.

I agree completely that the patient should have the opportunity of recording their conversation with the physician. I find that it is a tremendous emotional shock to a patient to learn that he or she has multiple myeloma. They cannot possibly recall all that was said during a consultation. It is absolutely essential that they have the opportunity to play the tape again and again at home. I might also add that I always encourage other family members to accompany the patient for consultation.

I enjoyed the consultation with David Weatherall. I liked

*that he could "Think for as long as he wishes before he speaks."
His comment "We know so little about how the body works" is
well worth the wait.*

The section Why Living Proof? *is vital.*

*The comment "Such is the complexity of cancer" is a suc-
cinct summary of the problem.*

*The statement of Souhami and Tobias that "treating
patients with cancer involves awareness of how patients think
and feel." We cannot emphasise this point enough.*

*Also Michael Gearin-Tosh's statement "be proof against
being* rushed to treatment" *is a most important concept.*

Why Living Proof?

1

If you have cancer, you feel that you are in the power of two worlds.

The first is the world of research.

In the news, on the Net, there is scarcely a week without some breakthrough or lead. And we read about new research facilities:

> Behind new brick walls in Germantown, Maryland, drills whirr and saws whine as workers put finishing touches on a laboratory unlike any ever built.
>
> By the azure waters of San Francisco Bay rises the steel skeleton of a new university research center.
>
> (*International Herald Tribune,* 10 February 2001)

The second world that patients have to face is meetings with a consultant.

Two people in a room.

Probably not by an azure bay.

Each of these worlds is, at the least, puzzling for a patient.

Let us look first at research. I am not a scientist, and I am not trying to give an appraisal of cancer research but a sketch of how the world of research appears. Thanks to the media, patients are now better informed than we once were, but I doubt if we are less confused.

President Nixon famously declared "war" on cancer in 1971 with an initial government allocation of $500 million per year. By 1976 this was $1 billion, and by 1996 $2 billion. There is also "the lure of gigantic profits through patenting laboratory processes" (Roy Porter, *The Greatest Benefit to Mankind,* p. 579).

Each of us, however, is more than ten thousand billion cells, a number that, as Nobel Prize winner Robert Weinberg writes, "vastly exceeds the mind's ability to grasp." And a high proportion of these cells—arguably all—have the capacity to over-reproduce and cause cancer. You can even ask a devil's question: why is cancer not more common?

> Given the trillions of cells in the human body, is it not a wonder that cancer does not erupt often during our long lives?
> (Robert Weinberg, *One Renegade Cell,* p. 3)

There is the Human Genome Project. We read that its aim is to analyse our genetic structure, and to catalogue and map all the individual genes in the body. The completion of the Genome is a new era of hope according to the press, and not just the popular press:

> The monumental advances in molecular oncology and in understanding the human Genome are leading to an explosion of new and novel therapeutic agents . . .
> (*Clinical Cancer Research,* February 2001, p. 229)

On the other hand, no less a figure than Axel Ullrich, Director of the Department for Molecular Biology at the Max Planck Institute, goes into print with:

Even now, results that hold promise of new cancer treatments are very, very rare.

And when asked about the completion of the Genome Project, he replies:

> What does it mean when we say that the human genome is completed? It is not completed. Three billion nucleotides, which is three times the size of the human genome, have been sequenced, but we do not have complete genes and the sequences have not been identified . . . the next step will take a long time and cannot be done by computers.
>
> (*The Lancet,* Oncology, 1 September 2000, p. 52)

You may read a sharp remark:

> In commercial terms, the return on our huge investment has been feeble: if cancer research had been a business, the shareholders would have sacked the management and changed the strategy long ago.
>
> (*Your Life in Your Hands,* p. 10)

This is by Professor Jane Plant, a professor of soil chemistry who was herself a cancer patient. Or you may come across a report of Dr. Vincent DeVita, the director of the Yale Cancer Centre and a former director of the National Cancer Institute: "Within 15–20 years, I think cancer will become just another chronic, survivable disease, much like hypertension or diabetes." Another leading figure, Dr. Judah Folkman of Boston, is also of the view that "we may be able to convert cancer into a survivable disease."

Sometimes later dates are produced for these achievements: 2025–50. There are daunting estimates of the next steps:

The technology of the Genome project pales in comparison to what is required for the next stage . . . "Scale is important because the size of the problem is very large," said Frank Gleeson, head of MDS Proteomics. "It's not for the faint of heart."

(*International Herald Tribune*, 10 February 2001)

But some writers put the costs in perspective. The US federal government now budgets annually $3.5 billion on cancer; also pharmaceutical companies spend in excess of $10 billion on research. But the National Institute of Health puts the cost of cancer in the US in 2000 at $180 billion: $60 billion of medical costs, $15 billion lost productivity through illness, $105 billion due to premature death. So major investment is not out of place in purely economic terms.

In another area of thought, you may read that scientists once thought there were 200 or so different cancers based on where they appear in the body: lymphoma in the lymph etc. But when cancers are categorised by their genetic abnormalities, the number is over 2000.

It is also a fact that fourteen out of fifteen new cancer drugs have been abandoned during clinical trials.

"What is Joe Public supposed to make of it all?" asks Mel Greaves. And even he, Professor of Cell Biology at the Institute of Cancer Research, London, does not offer an answer but, in his own words, "a flavour of the challenge ahead" (*Cancer: The Evolutionary Legacy*, p. 248).

Such is the complexity of cancer.

2

Let me turn to our second world. A doctor and a patient. Two people in a room. You and your consultant. No lack of complexities here, and horribly focused on your life or death.

I wish to concentrate on one complexity, which is the centre of my argument.

David Weatherall is both a scientist and a clinician. In *Science and the Quiet Art,* he discusses a case from his own practice, a brother and sister who have a rare disease that causes profound anaemia. Both have "exactly the same defect in one of the genes that controls the production of their haemoglobin," but there is a difference: the sister has no symptoms, while the brother is sick and needs transfusions.

After years of research, Sir David has found that there is another gene that the brother and sister do not share and that helps the sister reduce her anaemia. This explains the difference a little.

But only a little.

"A little" is Sir David's own choice of words, and a significant choice. Why? Because there is also the dimension of mind. Unlike the sister who has no symptoms,

193

Often the brother is ill and cannot cope with life; at other times he manages to live with his disease and to function well. Yet he is always anaemic, and his symptoms are not related to changes in the severity of his anaemia. *In his case a more holistic approach—simply sitting and talking to him—uncovers an extraordinary saga*: difficulties at work, financial problems, breakdown of relationships with family members, and a host of other social problems.

As each of these is dealt with, the whole pattern of his illness changes for a while, and he is able to cope and lead a more happy life, until the next crisis.

After further delving, and only after talking to him for several years and slowly gaining his confidence, it finally emerges that many of his difficulties are based on long-standing agoraphobia, a fear of open spaces.

Thus what at first sight seemed to be a simple genetic disease turns out to be a complex problem, reflecting layer upon layer of social maladjustment set in the background of a completely unexplained and unrelated psychological disorder.

(*Science and the Quiet Art,* pp. 344–5, my italics)

Many languages contain phrases like "mind over matter" or "it is all in the mind," and these phrases are centuries old. Yet while the public agree that mind is important in illness, the idea is somehow too common to be taken seriously: we meet it as cliché in magazines and movies, and we let it rest at that. Or if we do try to think about mind in illness, the issues are so complex that we give up.

My argument is about temperament. Since mind is a part of temperament—the *ment*al part of the word temperament—allow me to start by emphasising the force of "mind over matter" in a very basic way:

It is well known that the suggestion especially by a doctor that a particular form of treatment is effective, can be very powerful . . . especially where the supposed benefits are reinforced by a caring physician who has built up a strong personal relationship with the patient. This . . . response represents a true biological phenomenon, possibly mediated through links between the central nervous and immunological systems.

> (Memorandum by the Royal Society
> of Edinburgh, House of Lords,
> Session 1999–2000, Select Committee
> on Science and Technology,
> HL Paper 48, p. 212)

The body's response to the mind is *a true biological phenomenon*. We move from psychology to biology. The move, if one wishes to phrase it as a move, is *"possibly* mediated through links between the central nervous and immunological systems."

It is a good deal more than a *possibility* according to the work of some scientists in a relatively new discipline called psychoneuroimmunology. In the words of Professor Candace B. Pert of Georgetown University School of Medicine:

> Recent technological innovations have allowed us to examine the molecular basis of the emotions, and to begin to understand how the molecules of our emotions share *intimate connections* with, and are indeed inseparable from, our physiology.
>
> *(Molecules of Emotion,* p. 18)

"A growing number of scientists," comments Professor Pert, see this as "a scientific revolution, a major paradigm shift with tremendous implications for how we deal with health and disease."

I shall return to this. For now we may associate the changes in David Weatherall's patient with "true biological phenomena" (Royal Society of Edinburgh) or "intimate connections with physiology" (Professor Pert): dialogue played a crucial role in therapy, and "the whole pattern of illness changes for a while."

Thus "mind over matter" is not an empty phrase. Folk wisdom is right to intuit the connection.

Why do patients hear so little about this area? They may hear more in the United States than in the UK, though not always from their consultants.

David Weatherall's patient, of course, lived long enough for the "more holistic" approach to have a chance. And Sir David made progress

> only after talking to him for several years and slowly gaining his confidence.

Here is a major problem. Doctors work under intense pressure. Where is the time? As David Weatherall has also written:

> the frantic pace of life in a modern hospital and the diverse technical skills required of young doctors in research laboratory, hospital, and community allow little time for thought or sleep, let alone talking to patients and their families.
> (*Science and the Quiet Art,* p. 329)

Talking to patients may get squeezed out. If so, what place is left for comments like these from a textbook on cancer?

Above everything else, treating patients with cancer involves an awareness of how patients think and feel.

> (Robert Souhami and Jeffrey Tobias,
> *Cancer and Its Management,* p. 4)

This is not psychoneuroimmunology, but it is a strong statement. *Above everything else.* Nor is it made by so-called "alternative" doctors. Professor Souhami is Dean of the Faculty of Clinical Sciences and Professor of Medicine at the Royal Free and University College London Medical School. Dr. Tobias is consultant in Radiotherapy and Oncology, University College and Middlesex Hospitals. For good measure, they have a combative section about what they consider to be "cancer quackery."

Their remarks point to the vital role of a patient's own thoughts and feelings, even in the context of the pressures of hospital life.

3

The title of my book is *Living Proof.*

Does the fact that I am alive prove anything?

No. Only that I am not dead. On the other hand, I would not wish to have done without my therapies, and I continue with them.

My point about proof is that the concept of proof is sometimes used loosely, as I shall indicate, and patients should view it with caution.

As a word, *proof* can mean not only *proof of* but also *proof against,* as in bulletproof, fireproof, soundproof, weatherproof, waterproof . . . This use of *proof against* comes from Shakespeare, who was a creator of language as well as of drama. The first use seems to be when Romeo says to Juliet in the balcony scene:

> *Look thou but sweet*
> *And I am proof against their enmity*
> (Act 2, Scene 2, lines 72–3)

There are enmities which cancer patients may wish to be proof against.

If you get cancer, you will be surprised how often strangers approach you for advice. Word travels somehow. I find that I am contacted once or twice every three weeks. Doctors may be irritated that patients consult each other, but the fact is that they do. Here is what I say.

Be proof against being *rushed to treatment*.

I take the phrase from a former Chief of Staff at Dallas City Hospital. Dr. Larry Dossey's life in medical practice leads him to believe that there is "a cancer mentality" that causes doctors to rush their patients into chemotherapy:

> The fact is, a cancer mentality exists among physicians, just as it does among the public at large. Cancer is currently the illness onto which, more than any other, we project our fears of suffering and death.
>
> In many ways this is irrational.
>
> Statistics show, for instance, that coronary heart disease is far more prevalent and carries a much worse prognosis following diagnosis than cancer in general. But most of us ignore these facts; it is cancer not heart disease, we fear most . . . cancer is a death sentence [we believe] and will end in terrible wasting and dehumanizing agony. Doctors often act out these dismal beliefs about cancer in various ways—such as by grimly rehearsing "survival" statistics to someone newly diagnosed; by rushing to treatment before the sun goes down; by exuding pessimism and doom in their discussions with patients and their families.
>
> (C. Hirshberg and M. I. Barasch,
> *Remarkable Recovery,* p. xii)

In my case, I was helped by a temperamental aversion to haste, an aversion I share with some of my heroes: I have mentioned Queen Elizabeth I's liking for "the hinder part" of her head, and Havel's wish to stay in "hibernation." Not fashionable positions. But if you are being rushed, ask your oncologist if there is a reason why treatment should not be delayed. Alas, urgent action may be essential, but in some cases, things may not be so bad. You may still be told that you have a "near pathological tendency to procrastinate," an historian's judgement on Queen Elizabeth I. I get told it often.

However, even in 2001, with all our advanced medical skills, diagnosis "may often be a surprise to both patient *and clinician*" (my italics). This is not a quotation from a lightweight source: the words are from the *British Medical Journal,* 24 March 2001, Volume 322, p. 730.

If you are diagnosed with cancer, you need time to think.

Perhaps your "surprised" clinician may also.

My next living proof is about thought.

Be proof against "proof."

Be proof against the concept of proof in the sense of being cautious if consultants bully you with it. If your consultant shares the spirit of David Weatherall, Professor Souhami and Dr. Tobias, you will not be bullied. Pray God this may be so. But the "cancer mentality" that Dr. Dossey identifies is, in his experience, widespread. It is not hard to find similar accounts. Simon Carr found that the manner of cancer doctors seems "to be designed to crush you into submission" (Simon Carr, *The Boys Are Back in Town,* p. 44). A Royal Society professor recently used the phrase "knee-jerk reactions" against alternative medicine: he deplored them, but the fact that he took the time to deplore them indicates that they occur (Select Committee on Science and Technology, HL Paper 118, p. 48). Equally, there are alternative doctors who crush their patients and deny the achievements of orthodox medicine.

What exactly happens in Dr. Dossey's account of the

physician with a "cancer mentality"? The doctor "rushes" the patient to chemotherapy on the basis of "survival statistics." The statistics are the doctor's "proof."

Yet what sort of concept is proof when applied to cancer?

Cancer research provides springboards for moving forward, real and significant springboards, *pace* the sceptics. Even so, for now cancer is still a "vast problem," write Professor Souhami and Dr. Tobias. They discern "progress" that they describe as "slow but steady."

The concept of proof is to be used with caution, if at all, in the context of problems that remain "vast." And what of the statistics that are the "proof" of "cancer mentality" physicians? "Even in the case of one specific type of cancer in one specific gender and age group," writes Dr. Catherine Zollman, an oncologist and psycho-oncologist,

> the best doctors in the world can only calculate average life expectancy.

The use of this is limited:

> Being told that a certain percentage of people will be alive, but that actual life expectancy could be anything from under two years to over thirty years, is of little practical help [for a patient].
>
> (*Integrated Cancer Care,*
> ed. Jennifer Barraclough, p. 282)

Allow me to bring together my two proofs: proof against rush to treatment, and proof against "proof."

I am not arguing that a "rush to treatment" is never vital. There is a warning to procrastinators like me in *The Precepts* of Hippocrates, written 2500 years ago:

> Time is that in which there is opportunity, and opportunity
> is that in which there is not much time. Healing is a matter
> of time, but it can also be a matter of opportunity.
>
> *(Precepts, I)*

There may be an opportunity for treatment, which must be taken at once. Miss it, and the chance is gone. You are dead.

I am arguing, however, that if you are being "rushed to treatment" on the basis of statistical evidence, this evidence may fall short of what you normally understand to be proof.

There is an interesting survey of cancer statistics by Dr. Ulrich Abel of Tumorzentrum, Heidelberg/Mannheim. Dr. Abel studied advanced epithelial cancer.

To avoid being technical, you may think of epithelial as referring to the cells that form the outer surface of the body and line the body cavities and principal tubes leading to the exterior, also the secreting portions of glands and their ducts. Thus cancers that originate in the skin or the lymphatic glands, some lung cancers and nearly all malignant tumours of the trachea, bronchus, stomach, colon, rectum, oesophagus, breast, bladder, pancreas, ovary, cervix, head, neck and liver are epithelial. According to Dr. Abel, epithelial cancers "are responsible for more than 80% of cancer mortality in the world."

Dr. Abel's studies led him to conclude that:

> Apart from lung cancer, in particular small-cell cancer,
> there is no direct evidence that chemotherapy prolongs
> survival in patients with advanced carcinoma. Except for
> ovarian cancer, available indirect evidence rather supports
> the absence of a positive effect.
>
> *(Biomedicine & Pharmacotherapy,* 1992, 46 p. 439)

Add the side effects of chemotherapy, and you can see why Professor G. Mathé of Institut de Cancérologie, Hôpital Suisse de Paris, wrote that "it is important to stop martyrizing patients with overintensive chemotherapy" (p. 435).

Dr. Ulrich Abel's paper was ten years ago. Statistics move on, and there are refinements to chemotherapy, but Dr. Abel makes points of general interest.

He observes that "many patients are treated according to uniform study protocols rather than to individual plans suiting their symptoms and needs" (p. 447).

"Many oncologists take it for granted," he writes, "that response to therapy prolongs survival, an opinion which is based on a fallacy and which is not supported by clinical studies" (p. 439).

And here is his conclusion: "It should arouse concern that according to opinion polls, many oncologists would decline to accept cytotoxic therapy in their own case" (p. 448).

If the proof of the pudding is in the eating, and the chef refuses to taste . . .

4

So far my two *living proofs* are negative: proof against rush to treatment, and proof against "proof." Is there a way forward? What about the word *living*?

What are you to make of the view of Dr. Catherine Zollman?

> the dominant healthcare system often makes the situation worse, not better.
>
> (p. 282)

Should you try meditation? Diet? Acupuncture?
All of them?
In combination with so-called orthodox treatments? Apart from them?
Is there a case for surgery and radiation, but for great caution over chemotherapy?
Is low-dose chemotherapy preferable to more "aggressive" chemotherapy? Should you avoid "overtreatment," a word used by Dr. James Le Fanu (*The Rise and Fall of Modern Medicine,* p. 352)?
Right?
Wrong?
There are no easy answers.

I wish there were.

The core of my argument is not "proof" but instinct, an instinct that there is gain in exploring questions about different therapies, if you feel you can. The gain is that you are more likely to become a *living* part of whatever therapy or therapies you choose.

Is there not likely to be a huge difference between active involvement in medical procedures, and what the poet and divine John Donne called "a rigid standing under an affliction" ("Sermon on Acts 7.60," 29 February 1628)?

It may be your fate to see consultants, orthodox or alternative, who behave like Gods. Simon Carr records how one oncologist said to Susie MacGillivray "you must have absolute faith in everything I say" (p. 44). But it does not follow that patients must share the depressed fatalism that such Gods tend to require. Simon Carr comments on the doctor who asked for "absolute faith,"

> considering the death sentence he was offering, you could not quite see the upside of doing that.

So what can a patient do?

The dramatist Arthur Miller has described the hold that Marxism exerted on his generation. It seems forbidding to apply his words to cancer, but they are a powerful answer to Dr. Dossey's "cancer mentality," to doctors who "crush you into submission," demand "absolute faith" or who give "knee-jerk reactions" in the phrase of the Royal Society's Professor Meade. Arthur Miller writes that:

> No one of my generation can be understood without reference to his relation to Marxism as "the God that failed," but I have come to think the phrase is wrong. It was an idol and

no God. An idol tells people exactly what to believe, God presents them with choices they have to make for themselves. The difference is far from insignificant; before the idol men remain dependent children, before God they are burdened and at the same time liberated to participate in the decisions of endless creation.

(*Timebends*, p. 259)

Doctors who "crush you into submission"—the Marxist parallel needs no elaboration—make their patients into "dependent children." Arthur Miller's alternative is to participate in thoughts about "creation." Creation can seem mockingly remote when you sense your own death round the corner—though not remote to a spiritual vocation, which asks us to see death as another stage of creation. Secular or spiritual, however, if your temperament permits, please give thought to Arthur Miller's paradox, fierce as it is, of being burdened and liberated.

Nobody opts for the nightmare of cancer, and liberation can be an impossible thought—too much suffering, too much trauma. But suppose your disease allows the thought. Recall mind over matter, and the "true biological phenomena" that even in the dry account of the Royal Society of Edinburgh can be "very powerful." Candace Pert calls psychoneuroimmunology "a scientific revolution with tremendous implications for how we deal with health and disease."

Professor Vernon M.S. Oh has commented that mind–body relations are "as clinically undeveloped as they are pervasive."

Alas that they are undeveloped in the clinic. Indeed, if your clinicians are not interested you may have to become your own clinic, as we will discuss.

But *pervasive* mind–body relations are. They work, in the words of Professor Oh, through

> largely subconscious interactions between the doctor, the treatment process and the patient
> > (*British Medical Journal,* 9 July 1994, 309, p. 69).

Here is the core of my argument.

Do you instinctively feel that a world of "largely subconscious interactions" is likely to trigger "true biological phenomena" on your behalf when you are "crushed into submission" to a therapy, orthodox or alternative, in which you do not believe?

Or do you believe that these forces are more likely to work if, to the extent you can, you are actively in favour of your therapy, if you see this activeness, however residually, as a participation "in the decisions of endless creation"?

You may regard Arthur Miller's phrase as grandiloquent in the context of cancer. And it is grand. But it may also be viewed in this context. Memorial Sloan-Kettering is widely regarded as the greatest cancer research centre in the world. Its president, Lewis Thomas, went into print with his belief that cures for cancer would "begin to fall in place at almost any time, starting next year or even next week" (*The Youngest Science,* p. 206).

This was in 1983.

What do you conclude?

That Lewis Thomas was a fool, and scientists are myopic? Or that the body is unbelievably complex? If the body is so complex, how about mind–body relations? "Emotions are indeed inseparable from our physiology," and with molecular evidence to support the view, Candace Pert and other scientists argue that there are levels at which there really is no distinction between the mind and the body.

(Molecules of Emotion, p. 196).

Even if you find it difficult to go so far in your own thinking, active involvement in your therapy may lead your consciousness and subconscious to trigger complex biological creativities, a presence in you of "decisions of endless creation" that may help to fight a terrible disease.

5

My experience is that among the major obstacles to this living involvement there are two forces that especially lower cancer patients to "a rigid standing under an affliction."

The first obstacle is puzzlement at the attitudes of clinicians, orthodox or alternative. When a patient does not understand something in a life and death context, it is easy to lapse into passivity. To be crushed. What chance then of subconscious involvement in decisions of endless creation?

The second obstacle to living involvement is a collapse of self-identity in another context. As a patient, you may feel that you have done what you can with your life, but can there be significance in your temperament and instincts when a world of zillion-dollar research sees your illness as "a vast problem"?

I plan to spend time over each of these two obstacles. Allow me, also, to note that the full phrase in Donne is "a rigid *and stupid* standing under an affliction."

Stark word, stupid.

But we shall have reason to use it.

Let us begin with the attitudes of clinicians.

You and your consultant.

Two people in a room.

When my friends ask about different therapies, more often than not they get attitudinising rather than argument. Dr. Knee-Jerk cries foul, fraud and quackery, Dr. Crusher goes puce, Dr. Wry knows of a clinic in Georgia that is closed half the year while its guru collects herbs. "Do feel that my door is kindly open after it all goes wrong for you," sighs Dr. Very Straight. Dr. Alert insists that if he does not see how something works, there is no point.

I exaggerate?

"His face dark red, spittle flying" as he "bellowed" disapproval is a description by Professor Candace Pert in *Molecules of Emotion* (p. 211). She describes an orthodox scientist, not a clinician, but they are the same when it comes to attitudinising. Beata Bishop tried to interest no less than seven orthodox doctors in her recovery from cancer after the Gerson therapy: she encountered contempt, anger, dismissal and, in her word, "bullying" (pp. 13–14). Of course, there are doctors to whom these strictures do not apply; I found wonderful doctors, as my narrative indicates. But allow me to probe the orthodox attitudinisers, "bellowers" and "bullies."

(It is not a part of my argument that comparable "bellowers" and "bullies" do not exist among so-called alternative doctors. They do. And they are a menace.)

There was a revealing episode in *The Lancet* that concerns what is now a mildly notorious editorial against alternative medicine. You will see attitudinising in print and in a high place: *The Lancet* is a top journal for the medical profession.

The context was Professor David Spiegel of Stanford University investigating patients with advanced breast cancer. Some received psychological group therapy, others did not. The aim of the psychology was to improve quality of life. To the surprise of Professor Spiegel and his colleagues, the psychology also increased length of life. Indeed, the average time of survival after diagnosis was doubled.

The extra life must have been a Godsend to patients and their families.

Double survival time.

Professor Spiegel submitted his result to *The Lancet.* The editors accepted it for publication but decided to write a tetchy editorial. They sensed, perhaps, that the methodology of Professor Spiegel was open to question, but they also worried that, although Spiegel was highly qualified, a study of such biological responses was close, as they saw it, to the fog that is alternative medicine.

The editorial opens as follows:

> . . . it is one of the central planks of the alternative medicine platform that mind can conquer matter and that the patient, adequately armed with the right attitudes of mind, can fight off the disease indefinitely. This line of thought invites one to define orthodox, complementary, and alternative medicine . . .
>
> Alternative medicine can be seen as the heir to the irrational and inductive schools of the past whereas orthodox medicine, if it prides itself on being a scientific discipline, must strive to be rational deductive science . . .
>
> (*The Lancet,* 14 October 1989, p. 901)

Let us examine the first paragraph:

> the patient, *adequately* armed with the right *attitudes* of mind, can fight off the disease indefinitely [my italics].

These are slippery words. *Attitudes*. Is not "mental discipline" or "mental exercise" a more appropriate term for the elaborate routines of yoga and for the Chinese breathing exercise in my narrative? The point is important since a phrase such as mental discipline points to wider issues: *attitudes* suggests that merely looking on the bright side is all that alternative medicine is able to recommend.

The wider issues are crucial to the word *adequately*. According to the alternative doctors who I know and read, diet, vitamins, physical exercise and thought all play a crucial role in therapy and would need to be included in a concept of *adequacy*. Note also that in yoga the mind is not separate from other disciplines such as diet. As B. K. S. Iyengar summarises in his classic work, the skills of breathing must be backed up by realising that

> Character is moulded by the type of food we take and by how we eat it.
>
> (*Light on Yoga*, p. 37).

In fact, *The Lancet*'s use of *attitudes* and *adequately* distorts and is reductive. It is not *a central plank of alternative medicine*, as *The Lancet* maintains, to isolate *attitudes of mind* where attitudes are viewed in a limited sense.

The *Lancet* editorial continues:

> The claims of alternative medicine will be readily accepted by the credulous because "belief is like an impression made upon the mind and that, the softer and less resistant the mind, the easier it is to impress something upon it." In contrast, the proponents of orthodox medicine must learn to be sceptical.

The tone is so like an uncle that you may scarcely notice the outrageousness of what is being said. Faith is only for *soft minds*? I shall return to this so-called rationalism and its arrogant self-congratulation. No matter that the editors express it in a quotation (from the Renaissance writer Montaigne); they chose the quotation.

The Lancet's main tactic is that *the proponents of orthodox medicine* are set against . . . who? Where are the proponents of alternative medicine? It is an old trick of politics to act as if the opposition did not exist. Or, to change the metaphor, you hold a court hearing but do not invite the defence.

The proponents of orthodox medicine are set against the *credulous*. The unspoken implication is that the case for alternative medicine is very weak: is there anything to be said for it that is worthy of a word like *proponent*? Alternative medicine? Soft minds, poor things.

Finally, in order to give the reassurance that comes from authority, *The Lancet* tells orthodox doctors that they "*must* learn to be sceptical" [my italics]. *The Lancet* is a professional journal for physicians, and they get a nip of authority. Uncle has standards.

Aha, what type of mind do you have, young comrade doctor? Stiffen up. You and I know that you are not one of those alternatives.

The editorial concludes:

> In this issue Dr. Spiegel and his colleagues in California report that psychosocial intervention can enhance the survival of patients with metastatic breast cancer. These results will undoubtedly reinforce the prejudice of all those who subscribe wholeheartedly to the mind over mat-

ter nexus—they do not even need to read the paper critically and their response will be "I told you so" . . .

Remember that *The Lancet* is a journal for trained, medical professionals.
So who are the readers who do not read critically?

Beneath this bluster, is it possible to find an argument?

Alternative medicine can be seen as the heir to the *irrational
and inductive* schools of the past whereas orthodox medicine, if it prides itself on being a scientific discipline, must
strive to be *rational deductive science* [my italics].

To avoid being technical, we will not go far wrong if we
see this as a distinction between what seems to work (inductive) and what can be explained (deductive).
This is a classic distinction in medical thought. You can
find it in *The Oxford English Dictionary,* which under *rationalist* cites this example:

Those physicians are called rationalist who do not value
the facts themselves so highly as their explanation.

Because the body is complex and so little understood, there
is often a gap—a gap of centuries, even millennia—between
observing that some remedy works (induction) and understanding why it works (deduction). The history of medicine
is full of examples.
The Lancet is right to argue that medicine "must strive" to
understand why cures and palliatives work, but it is prejudice
and a skewed use of language to call observation "irrational."
For example, people found out centuries ago that dock

leaves soothe nettle rash. Was it "irrational" to use them until dock and nettle biochemistry was understood?

And is there much difference between this and the "knee-jerk reactions" against alternative medicine that the Royal Society's Professor Meade deplores?

Is it not stupid—I use Donne's word—to knee-jerk the unexplained that works, because it is not yet explainable?

Yet the itch to knee-jerk is as old as recorded medicine. Hippocrates had to stand up for the importance of observing patients and for the fact that thought was involved in observing them. Writing in the fifth century BC, and with a use of the word "ancient" that takes us back well beyond that, Hippocrates urged his fellow doctors:

> not to despise the ancient art of observation *as if it did not exist* or because its method of thought falls short. We ought to admire the discoveries made by observation, and to realize that observation has made progress not by chance but because its own enquiries have been conducted correctly.
>
> (Hippocrates, *Of Ancient Medicine*, XII, 10–16, my translation)

As if it did not exist, as if observing patients actually did not exist: unless Hippocrates was exaggerating, he was criticising theoreticians who must have been as inflated as the Inquisition when it refused to look through Galileo's telescope because a system of logic demonstrated that the sun moved round the earth.

It is an irony that modern medical training emphasises the observation of patients, yet there is aggression against the inductive.

As if it did not exist: Professor Candace Pert writes of modern science that:

> Whenever something does not fit the reigning paradigm, the initial response in the mainstream is to deny the facts.
>
> (p. 162).

Allow me to conclude this section on a more technical note. Somewhere behind *The Lancet*'s attitudinising is a chestnut of philosophy, a question asked for centuries: is deduction superior to induction? The philosopher Max Black comments that:

> There is something absurd about the question—as there would be in asking whether the bricks or the beams contribute more to the building of a house. The fact is that formal insight [deduction] and inductive inference are not competing and mutually exclusive means for the achievement of the general aims of cognitive inquiry; on the contrary, *the conduct of scientific investigations constantly illustrates the need to supplement each process with the other.* It is a travesty of scientific method to suggest that much progress toward the discovery of comprehensive and systematic truth can be made without appeal to the formal disciplines of mathematics and logic [deduction]; but it is equally so to deny *the indispensability of induction.*
>
> We must remember that the high reliability of deduction is counterbalanced by the corresponding poverty of content of its products; induction may often be attended by a high risk of error, but the predictions resulting from its use are often of striking novelty and practical importance.
>
> (Max Black, *Language and Philosophy: Studies in Method,* p. 85, my italics)

6

I have taken time over *The Lancet* editorial because similar attitudinising and misrepresentations are heard in not a few consulting rooms, orthodox and alternative, throughout the world.

I now turn to the second pressure that can lower patients to "a rigid and stupid standing under an affliction." This is a collapse of self-identity, a feeling that your temperament and instincts have no place or value in cancer.

Remember Dr. Crusher, who "crushes you into submission"? He has patients who are *temperamental*—and, by God, he deals with them. But this is the only professional use he knows of the word temperament. "Can there be another use," he growls "in what our *Lancet* rightly calls 'rational deductive science'?" Thus orthodox Dr. Crusher. And alternative Dr. Crusher has no lack of other dogmas to invoke.

The value of temperament is that it is partly irrational. It is a mixture of the *ment*al and *temper,* instinct, passion, rage, areas we cannot articulate and where the semi-conscious may erupt.

Temper at its most vital was captured by the poet Yeats:

> *Even the wisest man grows tense*
> *With some sort of violence*

Before he can accomplish fate
Do his work or choose his mate.
(*Under Ben Bulben,* lines 33–6)

Even for the wisest people, there is a role in crucial life decisions for tension, violence, rage and the subconscious. Does anyone deny that fighting cancer is a life decision?

I return to Professor Souhami and Dr. Tobias:

> Above everything else, treating patients with cancer involves an awareness of how patients think and feel.

How a patient thinks and feels is, in part, a matter of temperament, and a crucial factor in all temperament, whether or not you have cancer, is how we regard proof, certainty and the unknown.

Are we frightened by the unknown? Can we live with it? Or do we pretend that the unknown does not exist? The poet John Keats made a distinction between those "incapable of remaining content with half knowledge" and the state of mind

> when man is capable of being in uncertainties, mysteries, doubts, without any irritable reaching after fact and reason.
> (to George and Tom Keats, December 1817).

I suggest that this is a relevant distinction to cancer.

No doubt there are a thousand points between the two states of certainty and uncertainty, and a few points beyond. But each of us has a position somewhere, although being such a complex lot, we are likely to have more than one position.

With regard to cancer patients, Dr. Catherine Zollman has gone so far as to write:

> For many people, being diagnosed with cancer is a bewildering and overwhelming experience, often the biggest crisis they have ever faced in their lives. Initially there may be waves of strong emotion—anger, fear, or sadness—but it seems that, of all the problems involved in coming to terms with a diagnosis of cancer, *uncertainty is often one of the most difficult to bear.*
>
> *(Integrated Cancer Care,* ed. Jennifer Barraclough,
> p. 281, my italics)

As a patient trying to understand myself and my fellow patients, I offer this thought: can Keats's distinction be of help? Uncertainty versus certainty. Is it possible to compare the temperament of patients in different parts of Keats's scale? Can we take a reacher "after fact and reason" and, on the other hand, a person "capable of being in uncertainties, mysteries, doubts"? What may we learn about each as a patient? Also, will we find a difference in how they explore therapies and view their own treatment, orthodox or alternative?

Is there a difference in how each type of patient might be a living proof?

The word *rationalist* will now feature in our discussion, and it should be defined. The rationalist reaches after reason, and there is a connotation that the rationalist's preference for reason does away with a need for faith. Remember, too, the medical use of rationalist that I have quoted:

> Those physicians are called rationalist who do not value the facts themselves so highly as their explanation.

This is also true of rationalist patients as well as physicians.

It must be added that the word *rationalist* refers to temperament and aspiration, not to skill. The rationalist *reaches* after reason, but it does not follow that the rationalist achieves reason, or achieves it in all contexts. A rationalist temperament in itself no more makes you rational than a musical temperament enables you to sing.

It is intrusive to move from generalisation to individual people, and no human being is simple: I am not suggesting that it is possible to categorise anyone's temperament except in very rough outline.

No cancer patient has documented their views as fully as John Diamond. On his death, *The Times* honoured him with an editorial that contained these sentences:

> He had as many hates as any columnist. They were mostly the rationalist's hates. He hated to be called brave since bravery was about choices which cancer patients did not have. He hated complementary medicine . . .
>
> (*The Times*, 3 March 2001, p. 25)

John Diamond is an evident challenge that must be faced by anyone who wishes to take further a consideration of these issues—all the more so since, as he wrote in one of his last articles:

> My one great pride in all of this is that there are now medical schools where they use the book I wrote about being cancerous as a textbook to give apprentice doctors some idea of what it is like to be a patient. What greater compliment could anyone pay me?
>
> (*The Times*, 24 February 2001)

What greater compliment could John Diamond pay to his fellow patients than to wish his prolonged suffering to give insights and to provide help?

I ask my questions of John Diamond the textbook, not the memory of a marvellous man. What is it to be a rationalist cancer patient? What is meant by a rationalist's hate of complementary medicine? Do cancer patients not have choices? Is there, from the start, a note of fatalism in this so-called rationalist position?

"He hated complementary medicine." I did not have the privilege of knowing John Diamond, but the word *hate* seems at odds with the love and humanity of his writing and of his life. So it should be noted that he also wrote "to be fair to myself I'm not quite the snarling sceptic I affect to be in print" (*C: Because Cowards Get Cancer Too . . .* , p. 98). Nonetheless, snarl or whatever, he was opposed to complementary medicine. In this passage he discusses why, and with less of a snarl than he used elsewhere:

> Here I was diagnosed as having a cancer which had originated no one knew where, a cancer which had a chance of killing me, and I was allowing people I'd never met to prod me and poke me and slice me up and subject me to dangerous rays following principles I didn't quite understand.
>
> How much better it would be if I could do something for myself, something based on some simple and obvious principle—that energy lines connect different parts of the body, that you are what you eat, that biochemical equilibrium can be reached by scourging the toxins from your skin—which would allow me to take control of my cancer. How wonderful it would be to decide for myself which of the dozens of equally valid remedies from around the world

was most suitable for my personality, my cancer, my birth sign.

I couldn't do it, though. I went for radiotherapy instead.

(p. 104)

It is impossible not to be moved by these paragraphs, and their tone is not simple. *I couldn't do it, though* is poignant and vulnerable more than disapproving. If there is a note of satire in mentioning therapies that relate to *my birth sign,* the satire is far from triumphant.

John Diamond thinks of his situation in terms of principles: surgery and radiotherapy were in accord with "principles I didn't quite understand," alternative medicine was seen in terms of "obvious principle." To this extent, he was a rationalising patient. *The Times* also wrote that John Diamond "hated the temptation to talk of higher powers," and a natural corollary is to reach for such order as may be found through the identification of principles.

The principles of orthodox medicine are those that John Diamond "does not quite understand," but he accepts his lack of understanding. To return to Keats, is this acceptance a capability "of being in mysteries"? Only in part, I think, and in small part. The main point is that doctors have gained John Diamond's confidence: so all is well, or as well as can be for him. The rationalist patient may accept authority on the grounds that doctors also reach after reason, and they do so on the basis of premises that are more expertly informed than a patient can hope to equal.

With regard to the principles of alternative medicine, John Diamond's attitude is different:

How much better it would be if I could do something for myself, something based on *some simple and obvious principle*

that energy lines connect different parts of the body, that
you are what you eat, that biochemical equilibrium can be
reached . . . [my italics].

Thus acupuncture ("energy lines"), diet and "biochemical
equilibrium" are based on principles that John Diamond is
confident that he does understand.
Why?
Because their principles are "obvious." He also finds that
the principles are "simple." Nor is this all:

How wonderful it would be to decide for myself which of
the dozens of *equally valid* remedies from around the world
was most suitable for my personality, my cancer, my birth
sign [my italics].

There are dozens more alternative remedies that John Dia-
mond has weighed up—we are not told how—and found
to be equally valid.
"Equally valid"?
Sometimes two approaches to a medical problem might
be called "equally valid," but it is unusual to find three.
Here there are "dozens" of approaches.
Twenty-four?
Thirty-six?
Forty-eight?
In fact, *equally* is a pointer that analysis has been left
behind.

What do we see in these paragraphs? Scarcely a rationalist
being rational: the premises of the argument will not stand
up. Are principles of diet "simple"? Is biochemical equilibrium "obvious"? Both are highly complex. Beneath the writ-

ing lies a collision between knowledge and the unknown, a collision that gives fear to all cancer patients.

We might ask what is meant by John Diamond's chosen criterion of judgement, the medical principle. Take his own example of radiotherapy. It could be called a principle that ionising radiation damages the DNA of a cell, and cell death will usually follow if the damage is not repaired. Radiate a cancer cell and it may die. But how far does such principle get you? It has to be put to work in the complexity of a human being, where "we know so little about how the body works." In this respect, it is like our earlier alleged "proofs."

John Diamond was told that

A burst of radiation will damage both [cancerous and healthy] cells but the healthy cells will recover.

Was it true?

"Well, up to a point anyway," he reflects, but:

it was with radiotherapy that I would first discover the principle of gradual disclosure which almost all doctors practise.

The principle is simple and at first glance makes a certain sort of sense. In the case of complicated, possibly fatal and emotionally charged illness, never tell the patient more than he is likely to find out for himself, and only ever give the best-case scenario.

In fact:

The radiotherapy turned out to have a mass of side-effects, it didn't kill the primary and it would lead to eight hours of major surgery.

(C: *Because Cowards Get Cancer Too* . . . , pp. 63–4)

•   •   •

"There is a terrible unfairness to cancer," wrote Liz Tilberis, and the unfairness hits each temperament in its own way. The rationalist "reaches for reason" but, as Roy Porter has written:

> despite the immense investment of money and research effort, cancer remains a disease *imperfectly understood,* in which relief is far more common than cure, and relief generally temporary and subject to serious side-effects . . .
>
> (*The Greatest Benefit to Mankind,* p. 577)

What type of weapon is reason against the "imperfectly understood"?

Yes, the world of orthodox cancer research produces hypotheses and supporting evidence that, in the words of Judah Folkman, may convert cancer "into a survivable disease."

In fifteen years?

But you have cancer now.

There is an "imperfectly understood" disease that threatens life in your body, a body of which, in David Weatherall's words, so little is known about how it works. The frustrations to rationalism are intolerable, and, whatever other factors are involved, the rationalist patient is in no mood to give quarter to alternative therapies.

7

The Times described John Diamond as rationalist: how far can we go in finding a non-rationalist patient according to Keats's scale?

As I look, I find that published accounts by patients incline to rationalism.

Helen Rollason "had to know exactly what a treatment is all about" (p. 35). Shortly before her death, she stated her basic stance in these terms:

> At the end of the twentieth century we're victims of the success of medical science—so used to the wonder drug and the miracle surgery that when faced with a condition that medicine cannot hack, we can't quite believe it.
>
> (p. 209)

Helen also had the rationalist's distance from religion. She was persuaded by an old school friend to go to Lourdes but spent much of the time "convulsed with laughter" (p. 83).

Liz Tilberis also wrote that "I'm not a spiritual person" (p. 130). She added qualifications about how her two adopted sons came into her life, but the centre of her stance on cancer seems to have been that she checked things out and "found the best doctors and entrusted myself to their care, their wisdom, their energy, and their medicine." (p. 279) The attentive reader of Liz Tilberis may question the extent to which she did check things out, and perhaps there is an element of disparity between *checked things out* and *entrusted myself.*

Ruth Picardie seems to have had places on both sides of Keats's distinction. She pressurised her oncologists but had "a lingering dislike of medication" (p. 31). On spiritual matters, as she wrote magnificently:

> Sadly, I am a Top London Atheist but death-bed conversion to Judaism not yet ruled out.
>
> (p. 35).

If the non-rationalist is elusive, is there a reason why? The psychoanalyst Adam Phillips has said that one of the things he "hates" about psychoanalysis is that: "Most people are essentially private and the demand to articulate oneself is quite often a real strain" (*Telegraph,* 7 April 2001). But at least rationality is verbal, and those who reach after reason have a spur to discussion, and even writing, which non-rationalists may lack.

As I search for a non-rationalist patient, I see why one of my favourite testaments in literature is a rarity. Non-rationalists may not write about themselves, but they can be written about by others. And this favourite testament of mine is a book where the writer was close to his subject and loved him.

Also both the writer and his subject were men of genius. A genius writing about a genius. Neither was a cancer patient, but, as it happens, both were ill. The testament is *Renoir My Father,* a memoir of Renoir the painter by his son

Jean Renoir, whose films include *La Grande Illusion* (1937) with Jean Gabin, Pierre Fresnay and Erich von Stroheim, and *La Règle du Jeu* (1939) with Marcel Dalio, Nora Grégor, Roland Toutain and, in the cast as well as directing, Jean Renoir himself.

I shall refer to Renoir the father and painter as Renoir, and to the son and film director as Jean Renoir.

This is how the book came to be written. Young Jean Renoir adored horses and joined a cavalry regiment in 1913. Early in the war, his leg was shot. Gangrene set in. His mother travelled to the hospital and opposed amputation. The leg was eventually saved. But the strain exhausted Madame Renoir, who had diabetes, and she died two months later.

Jean Renoir went to his father "who had not been able to walk for some years": Renoir had been ill with rheumatism for over a decade.

> The death of my mother had completely crushed him and his physical condition was worse than ever.
> (*Renoir My Father,* p. 9).

They spent weeks in each other's company.

Renoir was now seventy-four, Jean Renoir was twenty-one.

"Renoir took this opportunity to get close to his son," and these conversations form the basis of Jean Renoir's portrait, *Renoir My Father.* On its publication many years later, Jean Renoir wrote:

> I have often reproached myself for not publishing immediately . . . but now I no longer regret it. The passing of the

years and my personal experiences have given me a clearer
view of him . . . Now I know that great men have no other
function in life except to help us to see beyond appear-
ances: to relieve us of some of the burden of matter—to
"unburden" ourselves, as the Hindus would say.

(pp. 11–12)

There is little doubt that Renoir is in the non-rationalist half
of Keats's scale, and towards the extreme end. "What goes
on inside my head doesn't interest me . . ." he would say (p.
59). "When I think I might have been born into a family of
intellectuals! It would have taken me years to get rid of all
their ideas and see things as they are" (p. 17). Renoir liked to
put rational systems in their place:

Newton's discovery of the law of falling bodies is all very
fine, but that doesn't mean that a mother's discovery of
how to hold her baby isn't important too.

(p. 82)

"It was all very well for that fool Galileo to assert that the
earth is round and only one planet among others. Everyone
accepts this but no one acts as though it were true.

(p. 39)

As a young man, Renoir pretended to accept advice on
theoretical matters, and even to have been influenced by it.
But, according to Jean Renoir,

beneath the surface lay a blind unreasoning will. I might
even call it a subconscious will.

(pp. 288–9).

•   •   •

How did Renoir's "blind unreasoning will" cope with illness?

Seventeen years of illness, as it turned out.

He differs from my rationalist and semi-rationalist patients in that, for him, it was not an "important thing . . . to find a cure" (p. 311). He had been told that medical science "had not been able to solve the mystery of arthritis," but this does not stop patients—and cancer patients—looking for cures. The fact was, as Jean Renoir comments, that Renoir "was not a bit interested in his own health."

Renoir often said that he floated "like a cork." This attitude may seem passive, but his view of life gave a distinct character to passivity:

> He believed that our universe, despite scientific analysis and microscopes, was filled with mysterious forces. "They tell you that a tree is only a combination of chemical elements. I prefer to believe that God created it; and that it is inhabited by a nymph."
>
> (p. 132)

He sometimes called the nymphs fairies:

> Renoir was fond of fairy-tales . . . for him, daily life itself was a never-ending fairy-tale: "Give me an apple tree in a suburban garden . . ."
>
> (pp. 117–18)

These fairies were life spirits, and his passivity involved opening himself to the presence of forces in which he rejoiced.

Another of Renoir's attitudes was that he had:

no patience with those methods which attempted to extract more out of anything than it could yield . . . he did not like a *tour de force*.

(pp. 38–9)

Some cancer interventions may be called *tours de force*. The words of Dr. Dottino to Liz Tilberis were:

> Bone marrow transplant allows us to give an essentially lethal treatment . . . We take out some of your own marrow, freeze it in liquid nitrogen, and when you're sicker than shit, we give it back. We haul you to the brink, push you a little bit over, and then pull you back.
>
> (*No Time to Die*, p. 221)

To the rationalist, this is a triumph of human resourcefulness. The skills of science help you to stay alive, and they are a *tour de force* in the proper sense of the term, a triumph of ingenuity. But this is not how they look to everyone.

For the Renoirs, if I may generalise, it is not so much that the *tour de force* is against but apart from what matters. Newton and Galileo were not incorrect but they were "fools," too distant from the nymphs in the apple tree.

(Forget about what fell on Newton's head.)

If "daily life itself" is your "never-ending fairy-tale," you stay in touch with the trees and with the instinct which tells a mother how a particular baby likes to be held. These are sources of benevolence, and a living contact with them is your path ahead, which, you hope, will not lead to despair. But an "essentially lethal treatment"? It strikes an alien note. Are you not moving in the direction of the world of Frankenstein?

If it seems exaggerated to mention Frankenstein, you will find that some patients use this type of imagery. An example in print is Susie MacGillivray, who said of one doctor, "that oncologist . . . is a bloodless creep, he should be in some Dracula film" (*The Boys Are Back in Town,* p. 61).

"The modesty of true scientists is at one with that of true artists," reflects Jean Renoir, but outside that modesty, where "painters woo Nature, scientists violate her" (p. 395).

What of Renoir and alternative doctors? I wish I could balance John Diamond and his "rationalist's hate" of alternative medicine with Renoir liking it, but I have found no evidence. No acupuncturist comes into *Renoir My Father,* no precursor of Dr. Gerson, no equivalent of the book of folk medicine that Gerson was asked to read to his early cancer patient.

Renoir's therapy was work: "the more intolerable his suffering became, the more Renoir painted" (p. 398). Even on the morning of his death:

> He painted the anemones which Nénette, our kind-hearted maid, had gone out, and gathered for him. For several hours he identified himself with these flowers, and forgot his pain. Then he motioned for someone to take his brush, and said, "I think I am beginning to understand something about it."
>
> (p. 404)

As Jean Renoir remarks elsewhere, "I saw my father suffer absolute martyrdom, but I never saw him bored" (p. 40).

In the last years, it was his orthodox GP who not only looked after Renoir, but delighted him:

> My father said of Dr. Prat: "Just to see his eyes sparkling above his sheep-dog's beard makes me feel better."
>
> (p. 398)

Dr. Prat joins my list of hero doctors.

Of course rationalist temperaments may also work to their last day, as may patients who have received "essentially lethal treatment." And this non-rationalist position of Renoir has at least as many incongruities as the "rationalist" position that I have associated with John Diamond. It sits oddly with a valuing of daily life to "fume" against scientists while forgetting Pasteur and others who helped to keep more babies alive for the exercise of mothers' instincts. Renoir is disvaluing deductive thought as much as it was overvalued by those who irritated Hippocrates.

Daily life as itself "a never-ending fairy-tale" can mean seeing the magic in the ordinary. But what happens when the ordinary turns into tragedy? It is in fairy-tale as story, to state the obvious, that Draculas occur—or witches like Sycorax who put Ariel in a pine tree:

> Thy groans
> Did make wolves howl, and penetrate the breasts
> Of ever-angry bears. It was a torment
> To lay upon the damned . . .
> (*The Tempest*, Act 1, Scene 2, lines 287–90)

Susie MacGillivray's cancer made Simon Carr think of the agonies of Queen Victoria's ladies in waiting, who screamed from the pain of their tumours. I think of the newcomer to Solzhenitsyn's cancer ward who sees "a young man, thin as a rake but with a great bloated stomach" who "tore himself apart with his screams" (*Cancer Ward* i.i). And if Dr. Dottino creates a *tour de force* that can help, his *tour de force* is only possible because nature permits it. To quote Shakespeare again:

Yet nature is made better by no mean
But nature makes that mean . . .
    (*The Winter's Tale,*
    Act 4, Scene 4, lines 89–90)

There is small logic in calling unnatural what nature permits. In the words of a great biologist:

> if someone were to say that this course of action or inaction
> was the life that was authorized by Nature; that this was the
> life Nature provided for and intended us to lead; then I
> should tell him that he had no proper conception of Nature.
>   (P. B. Medawar, *The Future of Man*, p. 103)

8

A rationalist temperament.

A non-rationalist temperament.

(Neither of my examples is more than approximate.)

Why not have the best of both? We should try. It may help to save life.

Yet it is worth noting how temperament can be limiting. In *Confessions of a Philosopher,* Bryan Magee comments on atheistic humanism: it is especially common among the "able and intelligent" and

> tends to identify itself with rationality as such, and to congratulate itself on its own sophistication.

This self-congratulation is so pervasive that:

> Such people tend to take it for granted that anyone who adopts a different view from theirs does so from a standpoint of inadequate, or inadequately rational, reflection or intelligence—perhaps blinkered by convention, or religion, or superstition, or irrationalist beliefs of some more modern kind; or just plain muddle-headedness, if not thoughtlessness.
>
> (p. 200)

This is the stance of the *Lancet* editorial, it seems to me—not but what the Renoirs are also intolerant of what is uncongenial to them.

Doctors also have temperaments, as have researchers. "Emotions affect how we do science as well as how we stay healthy or become ill," writes Candace Pert (p. 21).

A doctor who is by temperament "incapable of remaining content with half knowledge" is a natural candidate for the world of deductive reasoning, while a doctor who is "capable of being in uncertainties" will find it easier, at least less irritating, to be more concerned with the oddities of observation.

Patients may wish to factor in the temperament of their clinician. As it happens, Chekhov wrote about seeing cancer patients with a colleague, Dr. Yelena Lintvaryova (it is in the Chekhov letter that Rachel Trickett preferred not to hear):

> [Dr. Lintvaryova] is an old maid, a quiet, shy, infinitely kind and loving, homely creature. Patients are sheer torture for her, and she is anxious to the point of psychosis over them.
>
> At our medical consultations we always disagree: I bear glad tidings where she sees death; and I double the doses she prescribes. But, where death is obvious and inevitable, my doctor friend reacts quite unprofessionally.
>
> Once she and I were seeing patients at the local clinic. One of them was a young Ukrainian woman with a malignant tumor of the glands on her neck and the back of her head. The malignancy had spread so far that any treatment was unthinkable. And because she was experiencing no pain then, but would die six months later in terrible agony,

the lady doctor looked at her with a profoundly guilt-ridden
expression as if to apologize for her own good health and to
show her shame for the helplessness of medical science.

(*To Suvorin,* 30 May 1888)

Is your physician a Chekhov or a Lintvaryova?
Was Dr. Lintvaryova "unprofessional," as Chekhov wrote?
She was trained as a doctor, not an actress. Her temperament
was how she was, and it influenced her approach.

9

Thus I have added two more living proofs.

Be proof against the impression that there must be more to clinical argument than may appear. My example was the *Lancet* editorial. You will often come across the elevation of so-called "rational deduction" over inductive observation.

The second proof is to be proof against a collapse of your self-identity, the reduction of your temperament to the merely temperamental. I believe that it is worth thinking about your own temperament in terms of how you respond to certainty and uncertainty. And you should note how pervasive temperament is.

These two proofs have an obvious connection. If you are uncrushed, if you remain yourself, you will be more alert to what Chekhov called the "dullwittedness and tyranny" to which patients can be exposed.

Chekhov wrote that:

Dullwittedness and tyranny reign not only in police stations. I also see them in science . . .

(to Alexei Pleshcheyev, 4 October 1888).

There is tyranny in the world of research science, and there is also tyranny among orthodox and alternative clinicians and journalists, a tyranny comparable to nothing less than a Czarist police station. And Chekhov was a doctor as well as a Russian who knew police.

I know of cancer patients who have been driven to despair, black paralysing despair, by attitudes and arguments that are little more than the tyrannising mindset of a contrary temperament, and that, if recognised as such, may lose some of their power to oppress.

Let us take acupuncture as an example.

I know cancer patients who want to try acupuncture but are cut short by curt consultants and by what they read. Allow me to take a passage by John Diamond. He had the grace to articulate his position, but, much loved as he is and powerfully supported, I believe that his position is wrong:

> Homeopathy has been going since the mid-nineteenth century, naturopathy for some hundreds of years in various forms; reflexology is based on principles and charts which pre-date most orthodox medical principles. Much the same goes for herbalism, iridology, acupuncture and any of the medical systems emanating from the traditions of the mystic East.
>
> One of the principles which is common to most of these systems is that *they have hardly changed from the day of their inception*; indeed many of their adherents take *pride in the immutability of their principles*.
>
> And yet until the early part of this century the percentage of cancer victims cured of their illness had remained more or less the same *since the year dot. Enter nasty orthodox medicine*, self-serving, arrogant, ignorant of lines of energy and pressure points, focused on the symptom rather than the whole

person, and what do you know? Suddenly people start recovering from cancer.

(pp. 103–4)

Do not let this type of argument prevent you from exploring acupuncture if you are inclined to do so. I believe that acupuncture has helped to save my life, and may do yours.

Some obvious points may be made about John Diamond's paragraphs. We do not have statistics *from the year dot.* Hippocrates did what he could with cancer, and Galen writes as if some of his patients recovered. But even if we did have statistics, *enter nasty orthodox medicine* begs two questions. The first is that there is more cancer now than in 1900, much more. Secondly, the early part of the twentieth century saw a dramatic improvement in most types of health care. Surgery entered a new era, helped by new antibacterial drugs, and X-rays were developed, as was radiation:

> Medicine was upheaved, revolutionised indeed. Therapy had been discovered for great numbers of patients whose illnesses had previously been untreatable.
> (Lewis Thomas, *The Medusa and the Snail,* p. 158)

But this was scarcely a cancer revolution.

Suddenly people start recovering from cancer: we may set John Diamond beside Professor Roy Porter and his statement that "lung, colon, liver, pancreas and other major cancers continue to have appalling fatality rates" (*The Greatest Benefit to Mankind,* p. 575)—this was written in 1997. Or consider Dr. Ulrich Abel:

> Today, many responsible oncologists are aware of the fact that strong evidence, both for a prolongation of survival

and for an improvement of quality of life by chemotherapy in advanced solid cancer is lacking . . .

(p. 447)

Turning to another aspect of John Diamond's paragraphs, is it true that acupuncture has *hardly changed from the day of inception*? The point behind his statement, I assume, is that the emperors of the Han dynasty (206 BC–AD 220) summoned acupuncturists as well as other healers, and ordered them to codify their knowledge. The *Yellow Emperor's Book* seems to date from *c.* 150 BC. On the other hand, just as Hippocrates pointed to "ancient" medical practice before the fifth century BC, it seems that acupuncture had been used for thousands of years previously. Examination of mummies and the Neolithic man preserved in ice, the Tyrolian Iceman,

> raises the possibility of acupuncture having originated in the Eurasian continent at least 2000 years earlier than previously recognised.
>
> (L. Dorfer et al., *The Lancet*,
> 18 September 1999, 354, p. 1025).

The date may be as early as 5200 BC.

The *Yellow Emperor's Book,* therefore, probably represents the advanced stages of a medical skill. Details of what John Diamond calls the *inception* of acupuncture are outside our knowledge. Why assume that acupuncture *hardly changed*?

Moving to the period of which we do have knowledge, Roy Porter observes with regard to insertion points that "the number grew" in the early texts (*The Greatest Benefit to Mankind,* p. 157).

My own acupuncturist, Dr. H., works cautiously within what he regards as an elaborate, if not exhaustive tradition.

Is this *pride in the immutability of principles,* as John Diamond
wrote? I see humility and observation of patients, not pride
in exposition of principle. I see a skill that is careful and conservative but also creative. Dr. H. has made a life-long study
of acupuncture, learning first as a boy from his grandfather
and studying acupuncture in addition to his extensive so-
called orthodox medical training. His acupuncture exem-
plifies what Halifax wrote: "the hardest thing in the world is
to give the thoughts due liberty, and yet retain them in due
discipline" (*Complete Works,* p. 237).

To conclude, as argument John Diamond's attack on
acupuncture is a house of cards. If science it is, in Chekhov's
words, science as tyranny and it should discourage nobody.
But are John Diamond's paragraphs best read as either argument or science? What of the biases of temperament? Note
the continuing presence in his thought of *principle*: the word
is used three times even in these paragraphs. What we find,
in essence, is a rationalist position. Deduction crushes induction. We do not know how it works: its advocates must be
soft-minded.

I wish to reformulate such arguments along the following
lines. We do not have much idea how acupuncture works. If
this distresses your temperament, acupuncture is not for you.
But if acupuncture attracts, you may note that it appears to
have remarkable powers, and has been thought to have
them for centuries.

In any case, it seems that we may be beginning to understand acupuncture. Some scientists mention enzymatic
pathways. And here is Professor Pert:

Acupuncture, too, looks very promising despite its having
been dismissed because knowledge about the points and
meridians, evolved over five thousand years of empirical

medicine, do not correspond to any existing Western concepts of anatomy. But absence of proof is not proof of absence. In my mind, meridians may be the pathways that are followed by immune cells as they move up and down an anatomical highway, a discovery that could be just one experiment away.

(p. 222)

Diet is another area where patients are often discouraged. And, yes, there are some cranky "alternative" ideas. But nutrition is an area that is increasingly explored by scientists, and its benefits are advocated by members, for example, of Harvard Medical School and UCLA:

> It is now appreciated that the process of cancer progression and metastasis may also be modifiable through nutritional intervention.

Or:

> the existing evidence of the impact of nutritional medicine on the quality of life of cancer patients cannot be overestimated.
>
> (George Blackburn, David Heber and Vay Liang W. Go, *Nutritional Oncology*, pp. 1–2)

Since my friends encounter so much discouragement from clinicians and writers—you may recall that "you are what you eat" was among John Diamond's "simple and obvious principles"—allow me to repeat that "the process of cancer progression and metastasis may also be modifiable through nutritional intervention." This is not of small importance.

Nor is the quality of life of cancer patients where "the existing evidence of the impact of nutritional medicine *cannot be overestimated.*" This is not crazy speculation but a matter of evidence.

Allow me to take a small example. Dr. Gerson made garlic a part of his cancer diet. John T. Pinto and Richard S. Rivlin of the Memorial Sloan-Kettering Clinical Nutritional Research Unit now write that "at least twenty garlic-derived constituents have demonstrated chemo preventative and therapeutic activities" (*Nutritional Oncology,* p. 401).

Induction vindicated?

Long live that neglected, if controversial delight, the garlic sandwich.

To conclude, in addition to temperament, there are issues of ignorance.

You may be one of those people whose temperament is at ease with so-called unorthodox possibilities, but you may also be crushed by a tyrannising consultant or writer.

Check their facts if you can, and examine their arguments.

Be a living proof against, in Donne's words, "a stupid standing under an affliction."

10

A last glance at my argument.

I have argued on the basis of instinct that subconscious processes of healing will be energised less by "a rigid standing under an affliction" than by a wish to participate "in decisions of endless creation." Instinct was my own guide, but subsequently I have read a small amount concerning psychoneuroimmunology.

There are scientists and clinicians who scarcely accept psychoneuroimmunology. Professor Candace Pert, whom I use as my authority, writes of "a paradox of scientific progress":

> Genuinely new and important ideas are often subjected to nitpickingly intense scrutiny, if not outright rejection and revulsion . . .
>
> (p. 19)

By coincidence, the word *rigid* occurs in Candace Pert. She does not quote Donne: *rigid* is her own description of the view of mind and body before psychoneuroimmunology, a view which is now outdated for her, although still "the reigning paradigm" in science. In this rigid view:

the old guard cling to a concept of the body as unintelligent, a bundle of mass and matter stimulated by electrical impulses [from the brain] in a more or less mechanical, reactive fashion, with little room for flexibility.

(p. 185)

As a replacement to this paradigm, Professor Pert argues that molecules called neuropeptides join the brain, glands, spleen, bone marrow and lymph nodes "in a *multidirectional* network of communication." Thus what occurs is not a command structure of direction by the mind, "rigid rather than fluid, even macho in its reliance on force and control" (p. 256). Instead, there is "a constant *exchange*" that produces "an intelligently orchestrated symphony of life . . . intelligence is located not only in the brain but in cells that are distributed . . . mind does not dominate body, it *becomes* body—body and mind are one" (pp. 184–7).

Our phrase "mind over matter" is a relic of the earlier paradigm, and should be replaced by expressions like "body-mind," words from China and the Orient where medicine has not separated mind and body, as in the West. Part of John Diamond's attack on acupuncture was to use the phrase "mystic East" in a more or less pejorative way: Professor Pert's research on neuropeptides indicates that there is substance to this so-called mysticism.

Professor Pert, in another coincidence between us, writes about David Spiegel, the Stanford professor whose work provoked the *Lancet* editorial on alternative medicine. Spiegel showed that being able to express emotions like anger and grief extends survival time. Professor Pert offers "a theoretical model to explain why this might be so." Emotional expression "is tied to a specific flow of peptides in the body" and their suppression "results in a massive disturbance of the psychosomatic network." Hence their release is likely to be beneficial.

Could a disruption of peptide flow also disrupt killer cells and cause us to develop cancer? asks Professor Pert:

> These are the sort of questions we have to start addressing if we take the links between body and mind seriously.
>
> (p. 192)

There are several other areas in which psychoneuroim-munology complements, or seems to complement, my argument.

The neuropeptide information exchange is subconscious on the whole. I find it interesting that Jean Renoir felt that only a phrase like "subconscious will" could describe his father's inner resilience.

David Weatherall's patient suffered from anaemia and also agoraphobia. To Sir David, the agoraphobia was a "completely unexplained and unrelated psychological disorder." Could the relation be in some way connected with a disruption of peptide flow? If mind and body are one, such connections are not unexpected.

With regard to disruption, Professor Pert asks

> Is it possible we could learn to consciously intervene to make sure our natural killer cells keep doing their job?
>
> (p. 192)

Is this not what happens in the Chinese breathing exercise of my narrative? As you imagine scenarios and hunt cancer cells, you are spurring on killer cells to "keep doing their job."

Finally, allow me to return to the centre of my argument, Arthur Miller's distinction between idols and gods:

before the idol men remain dependent children, before God they are burdened and at the same time liberated to participate in the decisions of endless creation.

Compare "decisions of endless creation" with Professor Pert's description of how information travels throughout the body:

> Every second, a massive information exchange is occur-ring in your body. Imagine each of these messenger systems possessing a specific tone, humming a signature tune, rising and falling, waxing and waning, binding and unbinding, and if we could hear this body music with our ears then the sum of the sounds would be the music that we call the emotions.

> (p. 189)

Professor Pert gives the neurological evidence for a biolog-ical dimension to Arthur Miller's phrase, and if we are able "to consciously intervene" in this process through breathing exercises or visualisations, are we not participating at this level in "decisions of endless creation"?

Also, even if the intervention is not conscious in these forms of breathing or visualisation, my argument is that being a living proof may activate subconscious energising of the healing potential of this wondrous body music.

11

I end as I began with two worlds.

The world of orthodox cancer research shows huge promise, creativity and brilliance, although it is still true, as Richard Horton, the current editor of *The Lancet,* writes, that "Medicine is as unpredictable, baffling, ambiguous, fallible, and absurd as it ever was" (*New York Review of Books,* 2 November 2000, pp. 48–50).

A chill comes when I note that cancer has been identified in dinosaur bones from the Jurassic period—yes, of Spielberg's *Jurassic Park*—which is more than 150 million years ago (Mel Greaves, *Cancer: The Evolutionary Legacy,* p. 11).

Like the human species, cancer is a survivor.

An endless survivor?

But there is hope, real hope, that research will win.

Please, in time for me. For all my use of so-called alternative therapies, I want the fruits of so-called orthodox research.

And if only the distinction could disappear: in the era of Hippocrates, as a scholar has commented, "there existed no 'alternative' medicine, because there was no official medicine" (Jacques Jouanna, *Hippocrate,* p. 43).

Mind you, as we have seen, this did not stop patients being overlooked.

• • •

My second world is a doctor with a patient.

A patient with a doctor.

What fine choices from both, and instincts and tact and love may be needed for a living involvement in treatment.

With no guarantee of success.

For now.

An article by life-long cancer statisticians ends by noting that the best information:

> seems to come to the most trustworthy professionals from years of thoughtful listening, from a genuine sense of caring, and from a quiet scholarship that emerges from having learned that there are many paths for dealing with this difficult disease.
>
> (Jeanne Achterberg and G. Frank Lawlis,
> *Advances,* Vol. 8, 1992, p. 4)

I am immensely privileged to be advised and tolerated by Christian Carritt, Dr. H., Tim Littlewood, Neil Maclennan, Ray Powles, Hugh Riordan and David Weatherall, doctors who are living proofs of this tradition.

It is through the heroism of individual doctors that such traditions survive—and the heroism of those, like Charlotte Gerson, who maintain their work.

Here is a note from *The British Journal of Cancer* for April 2001:

> There are too few doctors seeing too many patients in UK cancer clinics with the added pressures of throughput and cost containment burdening them further. Furthermore surveys in the UK and US have shown that psychiatric

morbidity and emotional burnout are almost as common in oncologists as in the patients they treat.

(Vol. 84, pp. 1011–14)

This is terrifying. As the authors of the note comment, "the magnitude of the problem identified by this study can not be overestimated."

Governments must provide the resources to educate more doctors.

POSTSCRIPT

Raymond Plant, Master of St. Catherine's at the time, urges me to state in one place my daily regime at the end of my narrative in 1995.

My book has now argued that each patient should explore their own way with their physician: what works for me is not a prescription for you. Nor will most people want to try what I did. Even my hero, David Weatherall, has a dig at Gerson enemas: he speculates that a visitor from another planet "might wonder at the sanity of a society" that could extol their virtues (*Science and the Quiet Art,* pp. 18–19).

My regime was essentially that of Max Gerson (*A Cancer Therapy,* pp. 236–48).

The main points are twelve freshly made vegetable juices each day, with supplements of potassium solution, iodine, thyroid, niacin and pancreatin and a daily injection of liver juice and vitamin B_{12}. Dr. Gerson prescribed four or more coffee enemas each day: I managed three on a good day. A castor oil enema every other day.

Dr. Gerson had strict views about diet. These are elaborate and should be read in his book.

My own experience is that the problem with this regime, contrary to expectation, is not the enemas, juices and supplements but the rigours of the diet. So many foods are cut out—all salt and sugar, all cooked fat, for example—that what we think of as Western cuisine is prohibited. You get depressed because you find that there is nothing to eat, certainly nothing "convenient." There was a real change when I found that I could devise attractive, permitted food. It was a turning point.

In addition to Gerson, I took chlodronate twice a day, as prescribed by Ray Powles, to protect my bones. I also took vitamin C because of the Pauling and Hoffer article mentioned in my text. I had built it up to about 9 grams a day.

Finally, no day passed without the Chinese breathing exercise, the elaborate bone by bone procedure that I have described, followed by visualisation fantasies. When I could, I did the exercise twice.

In China and in Dr. H, Asia was as present and precious to me as the West.

These are time-consuming procedures. You need a helper, and I was fortunate in mine.

You must also have the support of your employer. The Labour government in Britain has now declared that cancer patients should be supported in the workplace. I put on record that years before, the University of Oxford, Vice-Chancellor Peter North, my faculty and my college not only gave me support, but also the hope that I could come back and continue to work. In the years to come, this was a vital psychological uplift.

from Professor Robert A. Kyle (ii)
Mayo Clinic, Rochester, Minnesota, USA

Mr. Gearin-Tosh's discussion on the attitudes of the clinicians is important. I join him in disagreeing with the statement "Faith is only for soft minds." I have seen many instances over the years in which a patient with a strong religious faith has done much better than expected.

As a matter of fact, the patient who fights the disease does much better than one who does not. I have seen the latter literally "curl up and die."

In summary, Mr. Gearin-Tosh is indeed Living Proof.

However, I do not know what role the vegetable juices, supplements of potassium, iodine, thyroid, niacin and pancreatin, the coffee enemas, vitamin C, Chinese breathing exercise and acupuncture played in the stability of his illness. I believe that he had smouldering multiple myeloma that continues to remain stable. I suspect that his plasma cell labelling index and number of circulating plasma cells in the peripheral blood are very low. He may well have done equally as well with a nutritious diet and modest doses of vitamin C, vitamin E and a multi-vitamin tablet. I must confess that I personally have a good deal of scepticism about his programme. These therapeutic modali-

ties need to be tested in a prospective randomised fashion. If any of them prove to be of value, it would be important to know. However, if they are not useful, it would save the patient a great deal of inconvenience, effort and expense.

One does not know if acupuncture plays a role in multiple myeloma. It is effective in certain circumstances. I have seen acupuncture as the only method of anaesthesia for removal of a pituitary tumour in China. One of my colleagues (a Chinese neurosurgeon who is department chairman of a prestigious US medical school) scrubbed with the surgeons and stated that the patient had received no other medication except atropine pre-operatively.

There is no question that oncologists often reach for their chemotherapeutic agents when the pathologist makes a diagnosis of cancer. Multiple myeloma is very different. I have emphasised to our fellows, medical residents and students that if one is unsure about the need for therapy of multiple myeloma then he should withhold therapy and re-evaluate the patient in two or three months. In many cases, the patient has remained stable just as Mr. Gearin-Tosh. I had a patient with smouldering multiple myeloma who remained stable for 20 years but then died at age 93. I have also seen patients with symptomatic multiple myeloma treated with conventional chemotherapy (melphalan and prednisone) who have survived for more than 20 years. In fact, I reported one patient who was cured at 21 years when he died of cancer of the lung. Obviously patients who present with hypercalcaemia, acute renal insufficiency, skeletal involvement with fractures and pain, spinal cord compression, hyperviscosity or severe anaemia do need immediate therapy. I might also add that we do not treat the patient even if the plasma cell labelling index is elevated. The same is true for circulating plasma cells of the same isotype in the peripheral blood of the patient.

The advice of Queen Elizabeth I and Havel's wish to stay in "hibernation" are both well to keep in mind.

Michael Gearin-Tosh states that "However, even in 2001, with all our advanced medical skills, diagnosis may often be a surprise to both patient and clinician." The clinician is also pleasantly surprised to see the patient remain stable.

The question that no one could answer today is whether Mr. Gearin-Tosh would have done as well with no therapy as he did with the difficult and time-consuming regimens that he followed.

The goals of Drs. DeVita and Folkman to convert cancer to a survivable disease makes a lot of sense. If we could only convert multiple myeloma to monoclonal gammopathy of undetermined significance, we would have essentially defeated the disease.

This, however, is a big order.

How can we do it?

Many of us are looking for more effective chemotherapeutic agents, biologic intervention, etc., but the role of the "unorthodox" therapies in this case report deserve scientific scrutiny and study.

Carmen Wheatley's essay, The Case of the .005% Survivor, is particularly well done.

Her call for proof of diagnosis of multiple myeloma and the need for chemotherapy is correct. The diagnostic procedures for justification of treatment are needed just as is proof of "unorthodox therapies."

Dr. Wheatley makes an important point concerning improved survival in patients who have favourable risk factors. We must face the fact that patients who do receive an autologous stem cell transplant are pre-selected and, in general, have a bet-

ter prognosis than the average multiple myeloma patient. Patients above the age of 70 years, and those with serum creatinine levels >2 mg/dL, are not included in most transplant protocols. This will obviously improve the results.

Dr. Wheatley comments that "only time and further research with myeloma patients prepared to follow such eccentric protocols" may finally settle this question. We do need the appropriate studies to resolve this.

The precept of Hippocrates, "Primum non nocere" [the overriding priority is to do no harm], must still be kept in mind.

In fact, the advice of Hippocrates, "It is necessary to study all that one can see, feel and hear, everything that one can recognise and use," is still good advice after 2,500 years.

from Michael Gearin-Tosh

Professor Kyle and Sir David Weatherall are scientists and clinicians of great eminence; it is generous of them to comment on my book.

Professor Kyle writes that "the role of unorthodox therapies" in my case "deserve scientific scrutiny and study." The scrutiny may help other patients, and I am thrilled.

Professor Kyle considers it possible that I suffer from "smouldering myeloma that continues to remain stable." If this is the case, it may be noted that the smouldering was strong enough for my skeleton at age 54 to be that of a 90 year old man (see Carmen Wheatley in the essay which follows).

Not a kindly smoulder, and smoulder joins my list of words whose associations for the public are at a distance from their use in medicine.

One way of formulating the main question from a patient's perspective is this: have my therapies made a contribution to the myeloma remaining stable, and smouldering less?

THE CASE OF THE .005% SURVIVOR

Carmen Wheatley D.Phil Oxon

Foreword

This Case History has been written primarily for interested physicians, oncologists and Myeloma researchers. Well-informed lay readers should be able to understand Michael's protocols from this account—a glossary is provided on the Orthomolecular Oncology's website http://www.canceraction.org.gg, as are tables to which reference is made in the text.

The Case History has been peer-reviewed by Dr. Peter Gravett MB MRCS FRCPath of the London Clinic, Professor Ray Powles MD BSc FRCP FRCPath, Professor of Haematological Oncology, Head of the Leukaemia and Myeloma Units at the Royal Marsden, Sutton, Surrey and Dr. Robert Kyle MD, Professor of Medicine, at the Mayo Clinic. I would like to thank them all for their kind attentiveness, rigorous critique, and generosity with their time.

INTRODUCTION

"Multiple myeloma is incurable," the textbooks tell us.[1, 2] Median survival depends on the stage at diagnosis and can range from six months to five years.[3] Long term-survival is virtually unknown, but not quite. The 1992 survival curve for an unselected series of 156 patients at St. Bartholomew's Hospital shows a 2.5% survival at 10 years.[4] A much earlier study at the Mayo Clinic, covering 870 cases, found a not dissimilar total survival rate at 10 years of 2.2%, with a 3% survival for those 597 patients diagnosed in the 1964 onwards, post-chemotherapy, Melphalan era.[5] But among the 273 patients diagnosed in 1960–63, the chemo "virgins," there was only one 10-year survivor, a survival rate of 0.4%. This rare study of long-term survival in Multiple Myeloma observed 19 patients survive beyond 10 years, only 5 of whom were still alive at the conclusion of the study, one of these in his 18th year and 8 years out from standard chemotherapy treatment, still, miraculously, free of any evidence of Multiple Myeloma. Even the newer treatment approaches of high dose combination chemotherapy with stem cell support,[6] with or without alpha-2-interferon,[7] bis-phosphonates[8] or thalidomide,[9] have done little so far to

269

change the outlook for long-term survival and cure. In the world of haematological cancers, Multiple Myeloma is both at the most malignant end of the spectrum in relation to other B-cell neoplasms, and still the most elusive in terms of cure, though understanding of its molecular and genetic basis,[10] pathogenesis and management has vastly increased in the last decade, to a point which may shortly bear fruit, in novel, more targeted approaches.[11] At present however, the rate of attrition in this disease remains grim and undeniable.

CASE HISTORY

Michael Gearin-Tosh, aged 54 years, was diagnosed with Multiple Myeloma, IgG lambda, in June 1994. He presented with a chest infection, with "signs in his chest indicating he was suffering from bronchitis."[12] His principal symptom, severe night sweating, along with fatigue and some dehydration, led his doctor to investigate things further. Anaemia (HB 9.4 and mildly macrocytic), an unusually raised Erythrocyte Sedimentation Rate (125), and the presence of paraprotein in the serum (Table 1*), prompted a referral to a haematologist. A skeletal X-ray survey, electrophoresis and bone marrow aspirate confirmed a diagnosis of Multiple Myeloma (Tables 2 and 3), and it was proposed that chemotherapy with Melphalan be instituted immediately. The patient decided to take a little time to thoroughly consider the proposed course of action. At this point there was a second opinion, partly to ensure that a differential diagnosis of MGUS could be firmly ruled out,

*The tables and figures referred to in the Case History are not included here, but are available on the Orthomolecular Oncology website at www.canceraction.org.gg

and/or to ascertain the exact staging of the disease, since in pre–Stage I Myeloma active treatment can be reasonably deferred, sometimes for years.[13] In the event, in the months that followed, a total of three bone marrow aspirates were done (Table 3), and no fewer than four medical opinions were obtained at top institutes. (Fifth and sixth opinions on the basis of the extant medical data were sought in early September 1994 from Dr. Bart Barlogie, and Professor Sid Salmon. A seventh opinion was sought in early 1995 from Dr. Robert Brouillard at Scripps Memorial Hospital, La Jolla, California.) While the bone marrow aspirates are critical to a diagnosis of Multiple Myeloma, it is regrettable that not one of the three (or even the fourth done in 1996), should have included a Plasma Cell Labelling Index, let alone any cytogenetic investigation. The Bone Marrow Trephine Histological report notes the presence of "atypical plasma cells consistent with involvement by Myeloma," but does not go on to elaborate the qualitative abnormalities of these plasma cells. The first Bone Marrow Aspirate (Table 4) did not even specify the percentage of plasmacytosis, and yet, on the basis of this, the patient was, as he has phrased it, "being rushed to treatment." There is a paradox that should be noted here: on the one hand, less than meticulous diagnostic procedures are used to justify possibly life-threatening treatment. On the other, when it comes to the question of proof, as in the demand for proof of unorthodox therapies such as the patient eventually adopted, the medical establishment feels equally no hesitation in demanding Olympian standards of proof. From a scientific viewpoint, there is a certain inconsistency here.

Multiple Myeloma proceeds through a number of phases and stages: MGUS (Monoclonal Gammopathy of Unknown Significance), which is characterised by the presence of monoclonal protein in the serum, without other symptoms, and can last anywhere between 10 and 20 years or more,[14] corresponding to the latency period now acknowledged to be a feature of most solid tumours; Smouldering Myeloma; Indolent Multiple Myeloma; and Overt Multiple Myeloma, which in turn is divided into three stages (Salmon and Durie). Three haematologists, from the John Radcliffe, Oxford, and the Royal Marsden, Sutton, independently diagnosed the patient as having Stage I Multiple Myeloma. The patient fulfilled one major, and several of the minor, Salmon and Durie criteria[13] for active or overt Multiple Myeloma Stage I. The major criteria fulfilled by the patient was a serum "M" component of IgG >35 g/l: the patient's initially ranged between 37 g/l and 31 g/l at the second and third opinions. Subsequently over seven years, 8 out of 13 readings of his M component have ranged well above >35 g/l, up to a high of 45.3 g/l, and at the last record 35.4 g/l. Salmon and Durie Minor Criteria for Stage I Multiple Myeloma include a bone marrow plasmacytosis of 10–30%: (depending on site, the patient's ranged from 5–6%, "in keeping with remission," to 22%. This apparent anomaly in such a short space of time is a well-known phenomenon to diagnosticians, and merely the result of sampling at different sites, and focal manifestation. The higher percentage, from the sternum in this case, is the more meaningful one for diagnosis.) Minor Criteria also include an immune paresis in suppression of normal IgM and IgA immunoglobulins, which the patient had (Table 2); anaemia <10.4: the patient's HB was 9.4 one week before diagnosis, at which point it was 10.2 (Table 1); the patient also had diffuse myelomatosis though without apparent lytic lesions (Table 4). According to Salmon and Durie, one major and one minor criteria fulfilment is acceptable for a diagnosis of Stage I Overt Multiple

Myeloma, as opposed to just Smouldering, Indolent Myeloma, or MGUS. The patient had 1 major and 4 minor criteria fulfilment in total. At diagnosis, the bone loss was such that the patient had the skeleton of a 90-year-old man (Figure I). Diffuse myelomatosis carries a median survival of 31 months[15] and, in effect, the patient was told he could expect to live about a year and a half to two years, with treatment.[16]

Nevertheless the patient opted not to have treatment. What was his survival prognosis in this case? In the days before chemotherapy the median survival for Multiple Myeloma was 6–9 months.[5] This median survival, in the days before accurate Myeloma classification, may have included a few MGUS and/or Smouldering/Indolent Myeloma patients, so perhaps it erred on the side of generosity. The outlook could not be good. However, a certain stubborn optimism shared by both the patient and his advisor (the author of this paper) prompted the latter's curiosity on this front. During the two months that followed the initial diagnosis, while further opinions were being sought far and wide—from Barlogie in Arkansas, Salmon in Arizona, to Sherman in Columbia Presbyterian, to Powles at the Marsden—the question was put again and again: Did any of these clinicians have records or experience of long-term survivors, against all the odds? Surprisingly, now and again the answer came back: yes, there were outriders. If the clinician in question had been around long enough, an anomaly could sometimes be brought to mind. Dr. Sherman at Columbia had a patient *untreated,* and alive and well, with an "M" spike of 35 g/l, for over 15 years. Dr. Littlewood at the John Radcliffe, Oxford, could recall a woman who lived 20 years with Multiple Myeloma, though he had no explanation. The writer of this paper pressed Dr. Littlewood further: "What were the chances of anyone, let alone the patient in question, Michael, surviving 20 years or more, *untreated*?" Dr. Littlewood, after some careful thought, gave the answer: ".005%."

The pair of stubborn optimists looked at this figure unflinchingly. As hope goes, it was a very thin thread. But optimists never need very much to go on. If only one person had survived 20 years with Myeloma—not MGUS—untreated, then it must be possible for another patient to repeat this. There is always an outlier in most medical conditions. Dr. Littlewood, and others, offered hope: .005% hope, but that was enough. Though he will modestly tell you he is "just marking time," .005% at 20 years became the patient's survival goal. Having thoroughly investigated his options, he elected not to undergo standard conventional, or avant-garde medical treatment, in spite of the fact that no fewer than four good, independent oncologists, including Professor Powles at the Royal Marsden, Dr. Barlogie at the University of Arkansas, and no less an authority than Sid Salmon himself, the expert in Myeloma staging, on more than one occasion urged treatment as a matter of high priority. He did however adopt an alternative course of action with a strong biochemical rationale. Since the odds were so heavily stacked against him, it must be concluded that if such a course of action led to his continued survival and health, then it was not perhaps an accident, or coincidence, that the patient, who was supposed to have died within 31 months of diagnosis, *with* treatment, should instead be, nearly 8 years later, in that mysterious "plateau" phase so rarely characteristic of this disease.

The alternative course of treatment is worthy of consideration because it has almost certainly promoted this remarkable remission.

THE TREATMENT

Initially, the patient elected to follow the Max Gerson Cancer Therapy. Inquiries at the Gerson Institute (Bonita, California, US) revealed almost no Gerson experience of Myeloma and certainly no long-term survivors. This did not deter the patient. Myeloma is not one of the most commonly occurring cancers, though latterly its incidence is on the increase,[17] and cancer sufferers often have recourse to Gerson at too late a stage, or have been pre-treated with chemotherapy, which seems to impair outcomes. There was also a caveat from Gerson himself who clearly viewed blood cancers as more complex and difficult to treat than solid tumours: "Their metabolisms are much 'deeper' and more differently deranged than we see in other cancer types."[18] The patient's advisor thought that the Gerson Therapy needed modifying to suit the special needs of Myeloma—the Gerson Therapy was primarily devised for solid tumours, where its chief successes seem to lie[19, 20]—and that the Therapy also needed updating in terms of the substantial and ever growing current scientific knowledge of the impact of nutrition on the molecular basis of cancer in prevention, treatment and recurrence minimisation.[21] The Gerson Therapy is currently overseen by Charlotte Gerson, Max Gerson's daughter, who has courageously promoted and maintained the Therapy since the 1950s when her father died. However, she has made only a few changes to it. Max Gerson was a doctor, scientist and empiricist. He would almost certainly have assimilated the explosion of current knowledge on nutrition in cancer and carried on refining and improving the Therapy. (There has been disagreement within the Gerson Institute on this issue. Gar Hildenbrand espouses the latter view.)

The Gerson Therapy then was to be modified by the addition of the input of the fathers of "orthomolecular" medicine, one of the greatest scientists of the twentieth century, Nobel Prize winner Linus Pauling and his collaborator, Dr. Abram Hoffer.[22] As Pauling once said: "It is not enough for a cancer patient to receive appropriate conventional therapy . . . To improve quality and quantity of life, a regime of good nutrition is essential."[23] Also brought to bear was much orthodox scientific work on adjuvant nutritional therapy in cancer, a field which now has its own textbooks,[21, 24, 25, 26, 27, 28, 29] thousands of publications in peer-reviewed journals, and a growing consensus on profitable approaches, largely, but not exclusively, pioneered by North American doctors and scientists at prestigious institutes including Harvard, NIH, the National Cancer Institute, the M. D. Anderson Center, the Linus Pauling Institute, Stanford University Medical Center, UCLA School of Medicine, the Cancer Institute at Edgewater Medical Center, Chicago, clinics such as Cancer Treatment Centers of America, the Center for the Improvement of Human Functioning in Wichita, the Block Medical Center, the Simone Cancer Center, founded by President Reagan's oncologist, Dr. Charles Simone, to mention but a few. The burgeoning number of professional, scientific conferences on Nutrition and Cancer[30] also attests to the promise and integrity of this "new" field.

To the patient's advisor it was evident that some of the science and medicine behind the Gerson Therapy, as expounded by Gerson himself,[18] was outdated. Thus critiques of Gerson's Therapy based on the original rationale would be largely redundant.[31] More interesting was the empirical fact that some people clearly did survive on the Gerson Therapy. The evidence was in part anecdotal: both the patient and his advisor personally knew of such remarkable cases, some of whom had achieved notoriety in print,[32] and even included a practising doctor. There was also, moreover, published peer-reviewed evidence which, encouragingly, showed statistically significant survival rates for Gerson versus chemotherapy in two cancers which could rival Myeloma in ferocity and intractability to conventional treatment: ovarian and Melanoma.[19, 20] Since the patient was prepared for the rigours and discipline which the Gerson Therapy entails, it seemed a good base on which to devise an orthomolecular medicine programme which might radically improve the patient's general health and, by considerably altering the biochemical environment and micro-environment of the tumour, make it difficult for the tumour to thrive. The aim of the programme would, realistically, not necessarily be cure, but control. The patient should be able to enjoy good health and reasonable energy, enough to enable him to continue to live and work well. It is the same aim that Professor Judah Folkman has envisaged for his developing anti-angiogenesis therapy,[33] and indeed of a spectrum of novel approaches to cancer now in the pharmaceutical pipeline. Since the current kill-or-cure mind-set has largely produced "kills"[34, 35] with both cancer incidence and mortality on the increase,[35, 36] long-term control seems at the least a more humanitarian option.

Principal Problems Faced in Myeloma

Multiple Myeloma can lead to a number of clinical complications, several of which can be very difficult to deal with and can prove fatal. In August 1994 the patient had all the appearance of a very sick man, and among the risks he faced were:

1) hypercalcaemia, due to the heightened osteoclastic activity in Myeloma, which can in turn lead to kidney failure, coma and death;

2) paraplegia/quadriplegia, due to potential vertebral compression fracture, since the patient was already 34.1 mg/cc below the fracture threshold of 110 with a 56% bone density, as a percentage of average bone density for a male age-matched control (Figure 1);

3) serious infections, such as streptococcus pneumoniae, s. haemophilus, Gram-negative organisms and staphylococcus aureus, which might lead to septicaemia, due to the fact that in Myeloma the humoral arm of the immune system is in effect largely deactivated, so that only cell-mediated immunity is left.

Any of these major problems can considerably shorten life in Myeloma. In addition to running these risks, the patient continued somewhat dehydrated, which suggested some kidney involvement and dysfunction (his urea and creatinine values were at the high end of normal—Table 1), anaemic and low in energy—the anaemia in Myeloma is thought to be consequent on bone marrow suppression and possible haemolysis by the tumour[37]—with continued night sweats. Therefore his proposed treatment would have to try and address all the above considerations.

TREATMENT I: THE GERSON THERAPY

The patient began the Gerson Therapy in the last week of August 1994. The therapy is composed in part of a diet which is largely vegetarian and low in protein, particularly so in the first two months when no animal or dairy products are allowed. The diet must be fresh—no processed food or additives; high-raw—salads, fresh fruit and juices—with only a small percentage of cooked foods, slow cooked, without water, to minimise nutrient loss. Finally, all ingredients must be organic to minimise stress on the liver, already compromised in cancer, by preventing the introduction of pesticides, preservatives and other toxins which might further promote carcinogenesis. We now know that some phytochemicals, however "natural" and organic, can be liver-toxic in varying degrees. Gerson seems to have intuited this and experimented so that the diet tends to avoid them; he issued a list of forbidden fruit and vegetables, pulses, sprouts etc. Instead, the diet highlights a number of foods in which modern research has identified some key cancer-fighting components: linseed or flax-seed oil—the Omega-3 essential fatty acids in this can interfere with cachexia,[38] being key components of the body's anti-inflammatory response, they oppose the bad eicosanoids which promote the lethal cascade of excess cytokine release in cancer, including Tumour Necrosis Factor and Interleukin-6. Omega-3 fatty acids also appear to interfere with metastasis and promote apoptosis.[39, 40] Indeed so impressive is the animal work demonstrating increased long-term survival in cancer with Omega-3 fatty acids, that the National Cancer Institute has already undertaken a trial of Omega-3s in breast cancer.[41, 42]

Gerson's key list of fruits includes apples, apricots, bananas, cherries, currants, grapes, grapefruit, mangoes, melons, oranges, peaches, pears, plums, tangerines. Apart from their well-known vitamin- and mineral-rich status, many of these fruits are rich in bioflavonoids. Black grapes, for instance, contain anthocyanins which have been demonstrated to increase survival in tumour-implanted animals;[43] apples contain flavonids such as myricetin and quercetin; the white rind in citrus fruit is also rich in quercetin, a star nutrient in the nutrition-against-cancer field. Dr. Patrick Quillin of Cancer Treatment Centers of America has assembled some interesting data on quercetin in cancer.[24] Quercetin has "the potential to revert a cancerous cell back to a normal healthy cell, called prodifferentation."[44] Quercetin also induces apoptosis or programmed cell death in otherwise "immortal" cancer cells.[24] It inhibits inflammation by reducing histamine release[24] and reduces tumour-cell proliferation.[24] Quillin also refers to new studies which show that quercetin "may be one of the most potent anticarcinogens in nature."[45] Among the reasons for this may be the fact that quercetin "competes with oestrogen for binding sites, thus defusing the damaging effects of oestrogen" in breast cancer. Quercetin is also "a potent antioxidant." It "inhibits capillary fragility which protects connective tissue against breakdown by tumours," in angiogenesis and metastasis. Quercetin also interferes with metastasis by reducing cell aggregation or "stickiness." It "helps to eliminate toxic metals through chelation."[38]

This is just *one* component in Gerson's fruit list. When we look at Gerson's chosen vegetables, a similar picture of intuition borne out by current scientific nutritional research emerges. Highlighted Gerson vegetables are cauliflower and radishes, along with cabbage and broccoli members of the cruciferous family. Crucifers are rich sources of iso-thiocyanates, which can modify carcinogen activation by altering the metabolism of nitrosamines.[46] Garlic and the rest of the allium family also feature high on Gerson's list: a common volatile component of garlic, diallyl sulphide, is a natural detoxifier and has been demonstrated to be a strong inhibitor of cytochrome P450 2EI,[47] an inducible liver isoenzyme, known to be activated in hepatic, colon and head and neck cancers, and which can activate carcinogens, including nitrosamines, hydrazines and carbon tetrachloride. Diallyl sulphide suppresses oxidative demethylation by competitively inhibiting P450 2EI.[47] Selenium, for which the allium family—onions, leeks, scallions, chives—are also a good source, has been demonstrated to enhance DNA repair mechanisms,[48] which apart from cancer chemo-prevention may also be essential in switching cancer activity off.

Gerson's fruit and vegetable diet could be subjected to exhaustive analysis in the light of modern nutritional oncology research. One can go on . . . Resveratrol, a phytochemical in grapes, has been shown to induce phase II enzymes, such as quinone reductase, in the liver.[49] Phase II enzymes are the liver's detoxifiers and, as Gerson posited, efficient detoxification in the liver is essential in both the prevention and treatment of cancer . . . To summarize, however, the World Cancer Research Fund's Report for 1997 lists the following compounds under continuing investigation in plant foods as having proven or potential cancer activity: dithiothiones, isothiocyanates, sulfuropanes, terpenoids, isoflavones, protease inhibitors, phytic acid, polyphenols, glucosinolates, indoles, flavonoids, plant sterols, saponins and coumarins. Gerson did not have any of this scientific knowledge, yet, empirically, he devised a method which ensured that a large range of these compounds would be delivered to the cancer patient intact and in pharmacologically active doses: the intensive fresh juicing regime, with 12 juices daily, one every hour. The juices, which are "whole" juices in that the juicing method ensures virtually nothing is discarded, are also rich sources of vitamin E, carotenoids and retinoids for which an extensive literature and clinical work have demonstrated differentiating and apoptotic effects in cancer.[26, 50, 51] Both carotenoids and retinoids regulate gap cell junction communication.[50, 52] It is via the cell gap junctions that growth regulatory signals are transmitted. Since cancer cells have poor gap junctions and consequent impaired communication, their growth is deregulated. Carotenoids and retinoids can reverse this and thus interfere with their proliferation and growth.

The juices can be seasoned with a range of herbs but salt is absolutely forbidden. Modern research again suggests that, as Gerson believed, sodium can be a cancer promoter.[53] Gerson's aim was to reduce sodium imbalances by replenishing the body's stores of the Na antagonist, Potassium. The juices are naturally rich in potassium. But since Gerson reasoned that replenishment of the body's potassium stores took time, he added a 10% solution of potassium, with an initial dosage of 10 x 4 teaspoons in each of 10 juices daily gradually reducing over 8 months to a baseline of 6 x 2 teaspoons daily. It is possible that by altering this particular electrolyte imbalance for the better, Gerson was once more enhancing valuable cell to cell communication.

Other prescribed Gerson "medication" which the patient faithfully adhered to included (Table 5): Lugol's Solution—an iodine supplement; thyroid extract; niacin—300 mg daily in 6 split 50 mg doses and sublingually, to avoid the "flush" response; pancreatin—4 x 3 tablets daily; and injections of liver extract and vitamin B_{12}—100μg daily. Iodine itself has anti-carcinogenic properties.[54] Allied to the thyroid extract, iodine was intended by Gerson to strengthen and normalise the function of the thyroid gland. We now know that if thyroid function is deficient not only are all aspects of body metabolism altered for the worse but, critically in cancer, the immune system functions less than optimally.[55] Conventional medical methods of treating cancer—chemo, radiation—routinely wipe out an already depressed immune system and do little to restore it. Yet, as Gerson realised, it is the immune system which is needed to fight cancer, and therefore building it up should enhance chances of survival.

Niacin has a number of roles in cancer: it improves aerobic metabolism making tumours more accessible and vulnerable to internal destruction by the immune system or external destruction by cytotoxic agents;[56] niacin lowers both cholesterol and insulin-resistance,[57] both good things from the point of view of restoring the characteristically deranged metabolism of the cancer patient to normal; niacin also generates ATP energy via the enzyme co-factor NAD (nicotinamide adenine dinucleotide)[57] which is important given that much energy is uselessly lost and expended in cancer patients through the apparently redundant and futile Cori cycle, and the high demands for energy from the tumour itself which often leads to raised basal metabolic rates.[58] Along with niacin, vitamin B_{12} is the only other artificial vitamin supplement Gerson permitted, at least for the first 6 to 8 months of treatment. He considered B_{12} critical because animal data indicated it was "very potent in the restoration of all different tissues, be they damaged by age, chronic illness, operations, degenerative diseases, intoxication or by other means."[18] Once again, modern science has corroborated this view: B_{12}-affiliated enzymes (the B_{12} molecule structure was only elucidated by Dorothy Hodgkin about the time of Gerson's death) have been described by chemists as "the ultimate radical cages and ultimate radical traps."[59] Moreover, B_{12} is now known to be involved in DNA synthesis, repair and methylation.[60] (Cancer cells tend to be hypo-methylated.) As a methyl donor for the enzyme methionine synthase, B_{12} is also crucial to the bio-availability of folate: without a good store of B_{12} in the liver, folate becomes trapped and much of the anti-cancer benefits of the intense folate concentration of Gerson's green juices would be lost. (Our patient characteristically made these juices greener than green by regularly incorporating in them dandelion leaves, nettles, wild herbs, which he regularly gathers from the Oxford marshes and his native Scottish hills.)

The last and most controversial[30] part of the Gerson Therapy is the use of daily coffee enemas, as many as four a day to begin with. Coffee enemas, which one might be humorously tempted to dismiss as a Germanic idiosyncrasy, had medical acceptance and respectability in the Merck Manual until the 1970s. Their day may yet return, since they are also a key element of Kelley's Metabolic Typing Therapy, as championed by Dr. Nicholas Gonzalez and currently in large Phase III trials for pancreatic cancer at Columbia Presbyterian Medical School under the auspices of NIH. (NIH has given Dr. Gonzalez significant funding for this trial, since he had already demonstrated remarkable survival numbered in years for this cancer, which is so lethal it kills in weeks or months at best.) Gerson's rationale for the importance of coffee enemas was simple: as the Therapy began to restore the whole biochemical environment of the tumour in the body, the tumour was liable to be attacked by the newly primed immune system and rapidly broken down to cause what we now know as "tumour lysis syndrome," a dangerous state of affairs which, if unrelieved, can lead to coma and death due to the accumulation of toxic by-products of the breakdown. Coffee enemas effectively avoid this by stimulating the liver's detoxification systems. Once again, Gerson has been proved right in this claim. Coffee enemas appear to stimulate the activation of the glutathione-S-transferase Phase II enzymes which catalyse the conjugation reactions of xenobiotics with glutathione.[61] (Of course, certain fruit and vegetable components such as the isothiocyanates in crucifers and naringen in grapefruit can also induce GSTs, so that detoxification in Gerson is not exclusive to coffee enemas.) The active ingredients in coffee enemas appear to be kahweol and cafestol, the palmitate constituent of green coffee beans. Recent clinical trials have demonstrated that coffee enemas also make a significant difference to late-stage pain control in cancer, reducing the need for opiates.[31] Since pain control in cancer remains an enduring problem, this is in itself remarkable.

The patient had no problem adhering to Gerson's prescription for coffee enemas, and during the first year regularly did 3 to 4 a day. Subsequently he cut down to a maintenance enema of 1 a day, only increasing this in times of stress or minor illness, when he claimed it made him feel physically better. This regime he has followed to the present day. Moreover, though Gerson prescribed an average length of 18 months to two years for the duration of his Therapy, the patient has made only one concession in gradually tapering down the number of juices to 4 a day from 1999 onwards. Otherwise, quite simply, he has never stopped.

TREATMENT II: ORTHOMOLECULAR ONCOLOGY

"Le terrain: c'est tout," said Pasteur on his deathbed. It is a guiding principle of nutritional oncology that cancer initiates and flourishes primarily in an environment, the body, which is both genetically and biochemically favourable. Moreover, the cancer process has the ability to further change, degrade and adapt the biochemical environment to its advantage. Nutritional, or orthomolecular, oncology proposes that in order to fight cancer successfully it is not enough to treat symptoms with surgery and cytotoxic treatments. Tumour burden should be lowered, ideally, by the least harmful means. Next, not only should the general biochemical environment be assessed and supported with the use of diet, supplements, and other biological response modifiers, but the particular metabolic derangements and adaptations caused by cancer should also be addressed. Cancer may then be checkmated. Of course, this principle is largely theoretical and hypothetical, based mostly on substantial *in vitro* and animal lab work, as well as epidemiology. Yet it is not exclusively so: since the pioneering post-War work of Dr. Josef Issels, whose "whole body therapy" at the Ringberg Clinic had a 16 to 17% cure rate for *terminal* cancer patients, more clinical evidence is beginning to emerge, at first anecdotal, but increasingly evidence-based, as in the NCI's "Best-Case Series," in retrospective and prospective studies and NIH-funded double-blind trials. There are also scientists newly interested in gathering and assessing systematic data on "Remarkable Recoveries."[62] A number of studies in this field again point to the central role of nutritional approaches. Dr. Harold Foster, for example, has found that of 200 such documented cases of "spontaneous" cancer regression, 87% used a vegetarian diet, 55% detoxification, and 65% supplements.[63]

Ideally, with this approach to cancer, treatment should be based on an assessment of biochemical individuality. In North America such testing is relatively easy to access. In

Europe it is still not routine; though a movement is afoot as testified by, for example, the existence of the excellent Paracelsus Clinic in St. Gallen, Switzerland, or laboratories such as the Medical Biolab in London and Health Interlink, a UK branch of the US-led Great Smokies Diagnostics. The Gerson Therapy makes few concessions to biochemical individuality, or indeed to differences amongst cancers (though serendipitously, its successes with Melanoma may lie in part in the fact that it is a diet low in L-Phenylalanine and L-Tyrosine).[64] Nevertheless, Gerson's is a cookbook approach to cancer. In the beginning, the patient's approach to ortho-molecular oncology was also cookbook, the treatment in general being gradually built up, refined and improved over several years, as information, time and resources allowed.

By the end of August 1994 the patient's advisor had conferred with Dr. Abram Hoffer and ascertained that, of the two Myeloma patients in his retrospective study with Pauling, one was still alive. (This study, done with terminal cancer patients, extended survival fourfold compared to controls.) The patient therefore started on the Hoffer-Pauling daily prescription, which was as follows:

Vitamin C (as calcium ascorbate)	12 g
Vitamin B_3 (niacin, niacinamide)	1.5 to 3 g
Vitamin B_6 (pyridoxine)	250 mg
Folic acid	5 to 10 mg
Other B vitamins	25 or 50 times RDAs
Vitamin E	800 iu
Beta carotene	25,000 iu to 50,000 iu
Selenium	0.2 to 0.5 mg (patient took 400 μg)
Zinc sulphate	220 mg (patient took 50 mg Zinc Citrate, which is more easily digestible).

Sometimes calcium, magnesium or a vitamin tablet.

This prescription was immediately modified by the patient's advisor who pointed out that individual high doses of particular nutrients can be antagonistic to other essential nutrients and thus cause imbalances and deficiencies. Therefore in orthomolecular nutritional treatment a broad base of *all* essential vitamins and minerals should be used. The American company Solgar's V-2000 (Table 8) was chosen as meeting this criterion, as well as because of the realistically high dosages across the spectrum. Anything not supplied in sufficient quantity, such as the Zinc and B_3, was then added over and above.

The impressive work of Cameron and Pauling in the Vale of Leven Studies[65] with terminal cancer patients and vitamin C (10 g oral a day), which showed an over fourfold survival time in the treated arm of the study, with a small percentage of unexpected cures, together with two dramatic case histories, one of lung cancer liver metastasis, one of brain tumours, cured in the first instance with 36 g of oral vitamin C daily plus radiation, and in the second with 36 g of oral C daily alone, were all brought to the patient's attention. He was urged to build up to somewhere near 25 g of oral vitamin C daily, in split doses. By June 1995 he had managed to build up to 9 g. In the subsequent year he went on up to 20 g, which appears to be about his bowel-tolerance limit. (As established by Pauling, the bowel-tolerance limit seems to be the measure of individual need, and can vary over time, as stress, illness and other factors demand.) The patient has remained on this dose of oral C ever since. Eventually, the patient also switched from calcium ascorbate, magnesium ascorbate, and Ester-C formulations taken in the first two years to straight ascorbic acid, since some authorities have suggested this form of the vitamin is more active.[66] (The pH of ascorbic acid is considerably higher than that of the stomach acid HCl.) Vitamin C therapy was intensified in late 1999, without altering dose, through the addition of 200 mg twice daily alpha-lipoic acid, which recycles vitamins E and C in the body. Alpha-lipoic acid is involved in the generation of ATP, and modulates both antioxidant and redox functions in the body. It is itself a powerful anti-oxidant, chelator and liver detoxifier and helps regulate blood-sugar metabolism.[67]

In late 1995 the pioneering educational work in ortho-molecular oncology by Dr. Patrick Quillin was also brought to the patient's attention. At the time, Dr. Quillin, nutritional consultant, writer and organiser of cutting-edge confer-ences in the field, envisaged an adjuvant nutritional formula for the cancer patient which would contain absolutely every-thing known to science to impact on cancer prevention and treatment, beyond vitamins and minerals alone. Shortly after this vision became a reality, in 1998, the patient adopted it and continues on it to this day (Table 9). (The beauty of Immunopower, apart from its all inclusive experimental aspect, is that it dramatically reduces the sheer number of daily pills to be swallowed, as most of it comes in powder form, to be blended with juices.) The Solgar V-2000 was then discontinued as redundant.

Other refinements and biological response modifiers added to the original Hoffer prescription (and now taken in addition to Immunopower) included: co-enzyme Q10 (200 mg twice daily; currently 50 mg once a day); L–glutathione, (500 mg daily plus 50 mg L-cysteine); folic acid (5 mg daily); E-succinate (800 iu daily); Maitake-D-fraction; peppermint oil (2 x 200 mg daily) and aspirin. Co-enzyme Q10 has a role in cellular energy transport and aerobic metabolism, as well as being an immune stimulant[68] and prostaglandin metabo-lism improver. Subsequently, Dr. Hoffer added Co-Q10 to his regime and noted improved results. L–glutathione is one of the most important and all-pervasive antioxidants in the human body, and it is invariably low in cancer patients. It is a key component of Gerson's favourite detoxifier, glutathione peroxidase. E-succinate, a synthetic form of vitamin E, has the ability, unlike natural vitamin E, the tocopherols, to actually work at the level of the chromosome in switching oncogenes off.[50] Maitake-D-fraction is derived from the oriental Maitake mushroom and its anti-cancer properties[69] have been researched and demonstrated to the point where it is used as sole chemotherapy for stomach cancer in Japan. Peppermint oil (200 mg twice daily) was added, and is continued with to the present day, because the attention of the patient's advisor was caught by a chance remark in a paper on the molecular biology of Myeloma to the effect that the menthol molecule is a match for the Interleukin-6 receptor. Since Interleukin-6 is overproduced in Myeloma and is the prime promoter of tumour progression,[11] it seemed sensible to try anything that might block IL-6. This was also the rationale for the addition of aspirin: aspirin blocks nuclear factor NF-κB, which is a key player in the production of IL-6.[70] However, the patient, being drug-averse, ultimately decided not to continue taking aspirin on a daily basis. So this was a short-lived experiment.

TREATMENT III: BISPHOSPHONATES

The patient's bones were a major source of concern. By February 1995, it was evident that the patient was doing well on his chosen course of treatment. Yet his bones, though stable, were not gaining density and he remained at risk of fractures and compression fractures of the vertebral column. The option of Bisphosphonate Therapy appeared to offer a double benefit, in that bisphosphonates not only interfere with the nesting of Myeloma in bone[15] but can increase bone density over time.[71] Intravenous administration with Pamidronate was discussed, but in the end the patient opted for daily oral Clodronate (dose 800 mg daily). This was begun in March 1995 but discontinued at the end of May 1995, due to recurrent intestinal upset, which the patient felt might interfere with the optimal absorption of nutrients from the Gerson Therapy.

Almost certainly, this was a short-sighted decision and an alternative route of bisphosphonate administration should have been sought. However, the patient continued with the bone-support supplements that had been started concurrently, namely vitamin D, and Dr. Vogel's Bioforce formula, Urticalcin, containing calcium, boron, silica and nettle extract. He also tried Novartis's Meritene for about a year, since this "nutriceutical" formula had been demonstrated in trials with wheelchair-bound elderly to halt bone loss by up to 50%.[72] The patient was told of the importance of exercise to stimulate bone growth, and chose regular walking as a safe compromise. In the circumstances, any more violent load-bearing exercise would have been too risky.

The patient's bones were regularly monitored (Table 8). In December 2000 it became evident that, though there had been no dramatic bone loss since diagnosis—the BMD of the hip remaining pretty constant—and there was absolutely no evidence of Myeloma activity, the trend for the bone density of the lumbar spine was going in the wrong direction, with a fall of 0.092 since July 1995. The loss could have been due largely to the natural loss of bone in age. But there was a more obvious explanation. A year earlier, in October 1999, a remarkable failure in the patient to absorb some of the key bone-building minerals was identified by

Dr. Hugh Riordan at the Bio-Laboratory, Wichita, Kansas. In 1994 the patient's advisor had intuitively suspected the patient might suffer from deficient stomach-acid production and had urged him to test for this. The test was not done. There was so much else to attend to. By 1999 the patient's continuing stability and good health were a fact. The question however remained: if the patient had had such a remarkable response to his treatment, why was he not continuing to progress? Why were the bones not gaining in density?

More information was needed. If progress were to be possible, the cookbook approach must be discarded. The patient agreed to go and have a state-of-the-art complete biochemical screen at Dr. Riordan's Center for the Improvement of Human Functioning (Table 9). The results of this should allow modification and improvement of his chosen treatment.

From the bone-building point of view, this screen revealed not inadequate calcium serum levels of 9.2 mg/dl. Levels of vitamin D were, by some oversight, unfortunately not measured. Serum phosphorus was off the graph at 5.9 mg/dl, which might suggest some increased osteoclastic activity. (This could also be spurious hyperphosphatemia, for which there are two possible explanations in Myeloma: occasionally the M-protein may bind phosphate,[73] causing a false increase in serum phosphorus levels; in IgG Myeloma in particular, the M-component can interfere with the phosphate chromogenic assay.[74]) Magnesium which, along with phosphorus, is essential in bone-building, was extremely low at 3.3 mg/dl; and the trace mineral zinc, also involved in bone-building, was also low, all in spite of supplementation. The latter deficiency might in part be "explained" by the patient's high pyrrole excretion. However, since supplementation of all the minerals was high, it must be surmised that the problem was primarily one of stomach absorption and a related deficiency of acid secretion. The utterly extraordinary thing was that, in spite of an important macro and trace mineral deficiency that had almost certainly existed for years, the patient had done so well on his chosen treatment. The brilliant adaptive powers of the body and its undeniable bent for homeostasis and health are well illustrated here.

The next logical step should have been a Heidelberg test or gastrogram investigation. This was not done until a year and a half had passed and the December 2000 bone scan made manifest the ongoing downward trend. There was now a sense of urgency and a need to gain a margin of safety for the patient on the bone fracture front. In late January 2001 Dr. Riordan prescribed Ipriflavone—600 mg a day, though up to July 2001 the patient mistakenly took 400 mg a day. A non-toxic synthetic analogue of vitamin D, "Drisdol," which can be safely used in high doses was also prescribed, and the patient takes 50,000 iu once a week. Ipriflavone (chemical structure: 7-isopropoxyisoflavone) is a synthetic isoflavone which has been demonstrated to increase bone density by at least the same percentage as bisphosphonates, if not more. Studies have recorded gains of as much as 6% in two years.[75] Ipriflavone, like certain bisphosphonates, also interferes with IL-6 activity and production.[75] It is also infinitely better tolerated, as well as having a better safety profile than bisphosphonates for long-term use. Ipriflavone is primarily anti-resorptive but also possesses bone-forming potential. It inhibits parathyroid hormone, vitamin D, PGE_2 and interleukin-stimulated bone resorption.[75] The mechanism of action appears to involve inhibition of activation of mature osteoclasts and further osteoclast formation partly through modulation of intra-cellular free calcium, enhancement of osteoblastic differentiation by expression of key bone matrix proteins and mineralization.[75] Ipriflavone does not have oestrogenic effects but nevertheless enhances the bone-building effects of oestrogen.[75] (Even males require oestrogen for bone-building.) Endocrinological imbalance in the patient was checked and ruled out in February 2001. Stomach acid levels and pancreatic function were then investigated, and the original suspicions were confirmed. Pancreatic enzyme secretion was slightly depressed, at 70% of normal, and HCl production was well below normal and classified as hypochlorhydria. (Figure 2.) The patient was prescribed between 300–1000 mg Betaine HCl before each meal. He elected simply to double at each meal his dose of "Acidol Pepsin," the Gerson supplement, containing pepsin 230 mg, raw pancreas 60 mg and Betaine HCl 260 mg per capsule.

At the end of June 2001, seven years since diagnosis, the patient also commenced bisphosphonate therapy with intravenous Ibandronate. Ibandronate is a 5th generation bisphosphonate with such a powerful dose-efficacy ratio, it need only be given in 2 mg doses once every 3 months. The Ipriflavone is being continued indefinitely alongside this treatment, and it is hoped that there will be a synergy between the two which, together with improved mineral absorption, will result in above average bone gain results within the next year. The patient is also fortunate in that this allopathic treatment, Ibandronate, is being administered by an orthomolecularly oriented physician, Dr. Wayne Perry of the Endocrine Centre, London. Dr. Perry will therefore monitor and adjust carefully all levels of calcium, magnesium and vitamin D, which can paradoxically be reduced by bisphosphonate treatment even though they are vital for its maximum efficacy. At present the patient has been prescribed "Calcichew D40" which contains 1250 mg Calcium Carbonate and 400 iu of cholecalciferol. Dr. Perry has also taught the patient a range of special exercises to help strengthen his fragile spine and promote its rebuilding.

Obviously, at the time of writing (summer 2001), the patient has a sense that he is on a tightrope: though his Myeloma is inactive and he continues in good health, the Myeloma might yet claim him retrospectively, through the initial damage done to the bones before diagnosis, damage which has as yet not been redressed. However, there are arguments that favour a more optimistic view. In spite of being well below the fracture threshold, the patient has had no fractures in 7 years of active life. Furthermore bone density may not necessarily reflect bone structure. It may be possible to have low bone density but relatively strong tensile structure. Dr. Wayne Perry remarks that he has seen far worse cases. There is hope, and the rational course of treatment now embarked on may soon well corroborate this.

TREATMENT IV: ENZYMES

Enzyme therapy in cancer is a controversial topic. There is considerable controversy as to whether enzymes can survive the process of digestion to reach the bloodstream in therapeutically efficacious doses.[76] Still, some intriguing claims are made, including the belief by Donald Kelley that cancer is the end result of a failure to produce sufficient pancreatic and digestive enzymes. Since Kelley's Therapy, which includes the ingestion of vast amounts of such enzymes, is now achieving some unheard of successes with pancreatic and other cancers, enzyme therapy may have some basis, and the various hypotheses[76] should be investigated further. One such hypothesis suggests that proteolytic enzymes act locally in the gastrointestinal tract to generate exorphins, and this would be of benefit since opioid agonists have anti-proliferative activity.[76] In animals, enzymes have been shown to slow tumour growth and metastasis.[77] In vitro, enzymes have been shown to both inhibit leukaemia cell growth and promote their differentiation.[78] The problem of enzyme delivery may or may not be a problem. The patient therefore decided to give Enzyme Therapy the benefit of the doubt. Of course, the Gerson Therapy is theoretically a diet rich in enzymes, due to its high raw aspect, and Gerson also prescribes pancreatin. The patient took the Gerson pancreatin until the end of 1998, and then switched to "Megazyme," a formulation containing 325 mg pancreatin, protease 81,250 USP, amylase 81,250 USP, lipase 6,500 USP per 2 capsules. The recommended dose of Megazyme is 5 capsules a.m. and 5 capsules p.m. The patient, however, takes 5 capsules a.m. only.

TREATMENT V: METABOLIC TYPING

In early 1999 the patient refined the Gerson Therapy further, influenced by Dr. Peter D'Adamo's book, *Eat Right For Your Type*. Dr. D'Adamo espouses the theory that individual blood groups reflect ancestral provenance. Particular diets would once have been characteristic of the individual blood groups as specific adaptations to the geographical location and environmental conditions of origin of these same individual blood groups. In his view, optimal health is achieved if you eat in harmony with your ancestral blood group diet. The patient is blood group A, for which a largely vegetarian diet with some fish is deemed appropriate, essentially the

Mediterranean diet, with olive oil high on the menu, fruit such as plums, figs, grapes, raisins, berries and pineapple, but in general no tropical fruits, such as coconut, mango, papaya, bananas. Potatoes, which are a staple of Gerson, are also banned altogether. The patient feels no hardship in all this. It seems natural to him. It should be said that Metabolic Typing can sometimes lead to prescriptions for diets high in red meat, and that this does not necessarily militate against successful cancer treatment, as demonstrated by Dr. Nicholas Gonzalez and Kelley's Therapy.

Treatment VI: Acupuncture

The British Medical Acupuncture Society makes the following statement about acupuncture: "Modern research shows that acupuncture can affect most of the body's systems—the nervous system, muscle tone, hormone outputs, circulation, antibody production, and allergic responses, as well as the respiratory, digestive, urinary and reproductive systems."

Research has also firmly established that acupuncture increases the body's release of serotonin, and endorphins, enkephalins, dynorphins and other natural opioids. Acupuncture is also thought to affect enzymatic pathways. Energy and mood can be improved by acupuncture. The corollary of all this is that acupuncture also affects the immune system for the better. No one claims that acupuncture can cure cancer. But its generalized effects make it a useful tool in treatment strategies that seek to alter the whole biochemical environment in cancer for the better, and optimise the results of other therapies.

This is the rationale behind the patient's use of acupuncture which began in September 1994 and has continued to the present, initially with an intensive regime of weekly, then fortnightly, then monthly sessions, and now at six-week intervals.

Treatment VII: Mind over Matter: Visualisation and Breathing Exercises

Mind over matter, like nutrition, is one of the oldest medicines in the world. As the 4000-year-old Indian *Mahabharata* (Santi Parva, XVI, 8 & 9), puts it: "There are two classes of disease—bodily and mental. Each arises from the other, and neither can exist without the other. Thus mental disorders arise from physical ones, and likewise physical disorders arise from mental ones."

To those who espouse the theological view that matter is mind incarnate, this is uncontroversial. Before the modern technological revolution in medicine, it was also taken for granted. As the great nineteenth-century physician and researcher, Dr. William Osler, said, "*Faith* in the gods or saints cures one, faith in little pills another, hypnotic suggestion a third, faith in a plain, common doctor a fourth . . . the faith with which we work has its limitations but such as we find it, faith is the most precious commodity without which we should be very badly off." Modern medicine with its stress on technology and allopathic drugs, largely forgot the power of mind over matter. Science, however, did not. The field of "psychoneuroimmunology" began with Hans Selye's studies on the effects of stress, and has gathered momentum and evidence at the end of the twentieth century with the work of George Solomon at Stanford,[79] Robert Ader and David Felten at the University of Rochester,[80]

Candace Pert,[81, 82] and Solomon Snyder at Johns Hopkins,[81] the very institute of which Dr. Osler had been a founding father. The contribution and connections between the mind, stress and cancer initiation and survival are now well validated.[83]

In devising a treatment that would capitalise on this knowledge, the patient was able to draw on both ancient wisdom, in the meditations and breathing exercises of Chinese Medicine, and the pioneering visualisation work of the Simontons.[84] These practices, begun within two months of diagnosis, enabled the patient to survive the trauma and stress of diagnosis, and the stress of life and work in general. The patient has given an eloquent account of these practices and the mind–body connection in health and disease. It is almost certain that, in terms of promoting a healing response, this was and is a critical aspect of his treatment.

CASE HISTORY CONCLUDED

The patient's blood chemistry and immunology results from diagnosis to the present show a picture of consistent and continuing stability of disease. Some improvements from diagnosis since the start of treatment are noteworthy. The abnormally high ESR rate of 125 mm/hr and 100 mm/hr at the time of diagnosis had fallen to 76 mm/hr by late November 1994 and one year out from diagnosis, in July 1995, was 36 mm/hr. The anaemia, which seemed to show some spontaneous improvement prior to commencing treatment, has persisted but remained relatively stable at higher readings. Albumin, an important index of nutritional status in cancer, which was low at diagnosis (30), has been consistently high in the forty-something range, with an anomaly of

34 in December 2000. Elevated liver enzymes at diagnosis also dropped significantly, and in general liver and kidney function has remained good. Lactate dehydrogenase, another marker for activity in cancer, also dropped from abnormally high levels of 352 at diagnosis and pre-treatment to a recording on the low side of normal, at 119. The blood count has remained normal, apart from a borderline neutropenia.

The results of the October 1999 Complete Biochemical Screen (Table 7) present a picture of a supremely well-nourished individual, with the above-mentioned exception of the glaring mineral absorption problem. Levels for all B vitamins are at the top end of normal, with Folate and B_{12} off the graph and, consequently, enviably low levels of homocysteine. The major antioxidants vitamins C and E are in the high, above average range, with a strong reading for A. The amino acid profile is very good, with one anomaly in undetectable aspartic acid, but conversely higher than normal L-asparagine, which may reflect low L-asparaginase activity in the patient.[85] (However, aspartic acid is usually only found in trace amounts in serum.) The essential fatty acid profile is also very favourable, with exceptionally low arachidonic acid, exceptionally high alpha linoleic, eicosapentanoic and docosahexaenoic acids. The monosaturate oleic acid is also at the top of the high range. C-Reactive Protein was negative. In tandem with this last, it is worth noting that the patient's B_2-microglobulin, like CRP, a major prognostic factor in Myeloma, has remained low over more than seven years.

So far the threat of serious infection has not materialised. In nearly eight years the patient has had flu once, three or four colds, the occasional stomach upset, an infected foot which responded well to antibiotics, and recurrent maxillary sinusitis, which is characteristic in Myeloma. This degree of infection is almost better than normal for the average healthy person, let alone a Myeloma patient.

As of July 2001, the patient is currently contemplating the further addition to his treatment of benevolent cytotoxic therapy, as exemplified by Dr. Hugh Riordan's experimental use of very high dose (50 g–100 g) Intravenous Vitamin C Therapy.[86] Dr. Riordan's institute has made a 10-year study of the use of intravenous vitamin C in cancer, and is now conducting Phase II clinical trials. Phase I trials were done at the University of Nebraska Medical School. This approach has produced remarkable remissions in pancreatic cancer[87] and late-stage lung cancer. The patient's rationale for using this particular therapy is that, as a matter of fact, the Myeloma is still in his marrow, however inactivated. Intravenous vitamin C can achieve a blood saturation in the order of 200% as opposed to 2% or so by the oral route. In vitro very high doses of vitamin C have been demonstrated to have an apoptotic effect on cancer cells. A method has now been devised whereby this can be achieved in vivo.[86] The hope is that just one final cytotoxic push is needed and the Myeloma will disappear altogether.

SOME HYPOTHESES FOR THE APPARENT SUCCESS OF THE TREATMENTS

A few general points may be made on the impact of the above treatments on cancer. Cancer initiation and promotion is known to be favoured by high levels of free radical generation that overwhelm the body's antioxidant defences.[88] The cancer process itself contributes to this imbalance, which in turn favours the cancer at the host's expense. It makes sense therefore to attempt some redress by supplying ample amounts of antioxidants, and both the Gerson Therapy and Orthomolecular Oncology do this, as amply demonstrated in our case by the patient's 1999 complete biochemical profile. Diets that are low in calories have been demonstrated to slow cancer progression.[89] The Gerson Therapy is based on a calorie-restricted diet. This is because it is very low in fats and simple sugars. (Gerson actually encouraged patients to eat as much as possible.) Another factor which can either promote or inhibit the cancer process is the body's acid–alkaline balance or pH. In the serum, pH is very tightly regulated (7.35–7.45). Elsewhere, in tissues etc. there is more latitude, though in terms of maximal enzymatic efficiency and health there is an ideal balance. Cancer is promoted by extremes of the acid–alkaline balance, but in particular by acidity. Solid tumours produce lactic acid, which makes their immediate environment more acidic. This in turn promotes their growth. It is not known for certain whether in Myeloma plasma cells do this in the microenvironment of the marrow. The patient's initially high lactate dehydrogenase levels at diagnosis, a product perhaps of cellular breakdown in the Myeloma tumour's environment, might suggest this is the case. (About 10% of Myeloma patients at diagnosis have raised LDH of more than 300 u/l.) However, the body's acid–alkaline base is important in all cancers. It is noteworthy, once again, that the Gerson diet and juices are naturally alkalising.

Angiogenesis is the means by which solid tumours spread and grow. Without angiogenesis there is no such possibility and cancer would be harmless. It is now known that non-solid tumours also rely on angiogenesis, in the marrow,[90] to increase in malignancy. This is the reason that thalidomide, an anti-angiogenic agent, is believed to be effective in Myeloma.[9] Interestingly enough, the primary impulse for

Pauling and Cameron's first experiments with high-dose vitamin C in cancer was the theory that it would act as an anti-angiogenic agent.[65] High doses of C would stimulate production of a substance that inhibits the enzyme hyaluronidase, produced by malignant tumours to attack the hyaluronic acid in intercellular cement, weaken their surroundings and allow infiltration. At the same time high-dose C would also strengthen the collagen fibrils in this intercellular cement, thus providing a double defence against angiogenesis. One might speculate that the patient's very high doses of vitamin C may, among other things, have played a crucial anti-angiogenic role in the marrow.

The singularly few number of infections experienced by the patient suggests that, though in Myeloma the humoral arm of the immune system is deactivated and/or depressed, what remains of the patient's immune system must not only be partially compensating but functioning optimally. In fact, the two arms of the immune system are far from separate and act in "a highly regulated feedback loop,"[91] so that some compensation is theoretically possible. For example, CD4 helper T-cells are usually involved in the stimulation of antibody production. If these T-cells are well primed they may be able to improve antibody response even in pathologically depressed states such as Myeloma. Conversely, it may even be possible that, since T-cells normally regulate antibody secretion through inhibitory lymphokine release, well primed T-cells may also be able to help regulate the *abnormal* antibody production in Myeloma. The treatments may have general immune system enhancing effects, but there are also some very specific effects. The integrity of lymphocyte function is dependent on good levels of folate. Natural killer cells, a subset of lymphocyte, are thought to be responsible for surveillance and destruction of neoplastic cell clones. This may be just as relevant to cancer remission as to its prevention. Folate, which the patient's therapies supply in abundance, is also critical in DNA repair and stability.[92] In Myeloma remissions, chromosome 13 remains stable, and there are probably no other genetic mutations or karyotypic instability. In order for T-cells, leukocytes, to function effectively they must be saturated with ascorbate.[93] Moreover high doses of ascorbate can result in greatly increased production of lymphocytes in the presence of antigens.[93] Large doses of vitamin C also boost production of interferons.[93] Some interferons have a known anti-cancer effect, Myelomas included.[94] Interferons also have anti-viral activity. Since synthetic interferons can be very toxic, Cameron's advice, "Take more vitamin C and make your own interferon!" seems sensible and is exactly what the patient did. Vitamin C is required for the synthesis of the Cl-esterase component of complement. Without vitamin C, complement is not activated. Higher doses of vitamin C result in higher complement output.[93] As there is some suggestion that complement also does not always function normally in Myeloma,[95] there is a rationale for supporting its optimal production. The complement cascade is, like a bridge, a critical part of cell-mediated, as well as humoral, immunity. Improving the function of complement may thus once more help in the compensation process that may have taken place in the patient. Pathogens that cannot be dealt with by complement are routinely dealt with by the widely dispersed macrophages. Macrophages in turn ultimately trigger the release of more complement. Of course, there are microbes that elude the defences of cell-mediated immunity and which are normally dealt with by humoral immunity. These are the dangerous microbes in Myeloma. Yet though in Myeloma humoral immunity is depressed, this is not the same as non-existent, and therapies which help promote a plausible compensation may well lead to a more efficient, if still depressed, antibody response, and therefore improved survival.

Proliferating Myeloma cells are characterised by an immature phenotype.[96] If Myeloma cells can be induced to differentiate into mature Myeloma cells, paraprotein production goes down, not up. The patient's paraprotein levels have remained more or less the same over 8 years. As noted before, both the Gerson diet and Orthomolecular therapy supply high doses of retinoids and carotenoids, which are used with success clinically, as synthetic drug analogues, to treat both head and neck cancers and certain leukaemias. Latterly, for two years, the patient has been taking a synthetic megadose vitamin D, for which there is also evidence of differentation potential in cancer,[97] as well as evidence to show it can promote apoptosis in Myeloma.[98] In particular, vitamin D is likely to work synergistically with the retinoids and carotenoids.

Overproduction of the cytokine, Interleukin-6, probably in a paracrine fashion in the humoral micro-environment of the bone marrow, has been established as the chief promoter of Myeloma cells' survival and proliferation. 500 to 5,000-fold higher concentrations *in vitro* and *in vivo* have been found for IL-6, as opposed to other known Myeloma growth factors: IL-10, OSM, LiF, G-CSF, SCF, IFN-∝(?), TNF-∝(?), IGF-1 and IGF-2. Thus current novel approaches to the treatment and cure of Myeloma are focusing on strategies for the control of IL-6.[11] Small trials of Anti-IL-6 monoclonal antibodies have been undertaken with some promise,[99, 100] and refinements in the pipeline include mutated IL-6[101] and humanized anti-IL-6.[102] But complete inhibition of IL-6 still appears problematic.[11] The test that is currently used to assess IL-6 inhibition is that for C-Reactive Protein, an acute phase protein produced by hepatocytes consequent on gp130 activation by gp130 cytokines, chief of which in Myeloma is IL-6. For this reason, lack of detectable serum CRP is also now used as an important prognostic factor, along with β_2 microglobulin, in Myeloma patients undergoing high-dose chemo and stem cell therapy/bone marrow transplant procedures. Unfortunately, the patient's CRP was not measured at diagnosis. However, in all likelihood it was present and possibly high, as indicated by his abnormally high readings for Lactate Dehydrogenase. However, in October 1999 the test for CRP *was* done, by Dr. Riordan, and the result was negative; exactly what one would expect for Myeloma in remission. This suggests that something in the patient's therapies was doing exactly what currently eludes scientists: completely blocking IL-6 overproduction and activity.

Induction of IL-6 is mediated by PGE_2, a key prostaglandin of the body's inflammatory response cascade. Agents such as indomethacin which oppose PGE_2 production also lower IL-6. A crucial aspect of the patient's therapy is the daily ingestion of flax seed oil, a rich source of omega-3 fatty acids. That the patient's resources of omega-3 fatty acids are at the top end of the high range was well established at the October 1999 full biochemical screen (Table 9). Omega-3 fatty acids form the basis of the body's anti-inflammatory response. If the anti-inflammatory response is good, production of bad eicosanoids and prostaglandins such as PGE_2 is effectively blocked, and levels of circulating cytokines, detrimental in cancer, such as Tumour Necrosis Factor and IL-6, are considerably lower. (A trial of omega-3 fatty acids in Myeloma would certainly be a much simpler and less toxic option than drugs which have still to materialise.)

Other factors in the patient's therapies which may have contributed to IL-6 blocking include vitamin C as a promoter of interferon production. IFN-α and IFN-β have been shown to affect MM proliferation, at least in part by down-modulation of the IL-6R receptor.[103, 104] Consequently, IFN-β reduces IL-6 dependent tyrosine phosphorylation of several signalling proteins which include RAS.[96] IFN-γ is thought to interfere with IL-6 transmembrane signalling, leading to enhanced apoptosis.[99] The patient's high intake of carotenoids and retinoids may also be a relevant factor, since it is known that retinoic acid induces apoptosis in Myeloma cell lines by once again downmodulating IL-6R expression.[99] As a general consideration the fact that the therapies appear to have boosted the patient's immunity, as evinced by his relatively low incidence of infection, may also be of relevance here. Infections equal inflammation which means high levels of IL-6 and CRP. Thus protection against infections may itself also protect against promotion and proliferation in Myeloma.

Critical to this discussion also is nuclear factor NF-κB, a transcription factor which is modified by redox status and regulates gene expression in inflammation and disease response,[67] including cytokines such as IL-6, and cell adhesion molecules. Myeloma cells secrete their own unique cell adhesion molecules which allow them to communicate with the bone marrow micro-environment,[96] and further their lethal effects. Furthermore, activation of NF-κB is also known to be a key factor in Myeloma angiogenesis due to its stimulating the secretion of such pro-angiogenic factors as vascular endothelial growth factors, basic fibroblast growth factors and IL-8.[96] Thus, once again, inhibiting NF-κB, which is usually dormant in the cytoplasm, may well be doubly beneficial in Myeloma. NF-κB activation occurs after

IκB phosphorylation and its proteolytic degradation, through extracellular T-cell mediated signals and/or Tumour Necrosis Factor-α, a rogue among inflammatory cytokines. Since oxidation is critical to NF-κB activation, anti-oxidants can play a pivotal role in its suppression; chief amongst these is α-Lipoic acid which, as we have seen, the patient supplements at high levels, not to mention all the other antioxidants the patient also takes. Aspirin, as already mentioned, also inhibits NF-κB activation but the patient ultimately declined aspirin. (However a trial of aspirin in Myeloma may be well warranted in this context.)

The above, far from exhaustive analysis may have begun to suggest some of the ways in which the Gerson and Orthomolecular Oncology therapies may work in Myeloma. The subject merits far more attention and research. Survival in Myeloma is so rare a phenomenon, and the exponential survival cure remains *so* immutable, that factors impinging upon it deserve to be scrutinised carefully for new clues towards achieving more successful treatment and cure. An open mind is a prerequisite of such scrutiny.

CONCLUSION

"Imagination is more important than knowledge," Einstein once said. Imagination is not usually mentioned in medical case histories. Yet it was the patient's imagination which opened up the closed world of a doomed diagnosis, and led to the discovery of other knowledge that has so far saved his life. The hallmark of the patient's survival has been the balanced interplay of imagination and knowledge, the exercise of impressive will-power, discipline and consistency. It is true he has also had tremendous backing from friends, colleagues and doctors. Whether he lives or dies, his is an awe-inspiring achievement. It is a medical achievement as well. By the statistical reckoning behind our representative opening study of long-term survivors, the patient, placed retrospectively in the non-chemo treated arm, for which one can draw up an asymptotic survival curve, would now, in year 8, have reached approximately 0.5% survivorship, bearing in mind that, in the days before chemotherapy, median survival in Myeloma was between 6–9 months.[105] The patient did not undergo chemotherapy, but did follow an alternative, unique and novel form of treatment, which no one with Myeloma has ever done before. In this study, in his class, he is a 100% survivor. Or 80%, if you take ten years as the goal. Whimsy aside, the patient's achievement can be put in a more serious context: the best results of medical advances in Myeloma to date.

Bart Barlogie at Arkansas and Ray Powles at the Marsden are two of the pioneers of the new high-dose chemotherapy approach to Myeloma with stem cell support and bone marrow transplant, followed by interferon and thalidomide treatment where necessary. Both Barlogie and Powles have shown immense dedication and enterprise in nearly two decades of this work. The patient investigated what both had to offer thoroughly before declining. This new approach is now well over a decade old. Barlogie and Powles have published numerous papers on results to date. They have been able to identify with some accuracy a defined sub-group of patients who will benefit from the new treatment. For this sub-group Barlogie and Powles have effected some apparent genuine gains: complete remission rates—50% and 48.4% respectively, and increased overall survival in the order of 4.9 to >5 years.[106, 107] These studies follow patients for more than a decade. In summer 2001 Powles appeared in *The*

Times with 2 ten-year survivors and cited a total of 14 ten-year survivors as a result of his work. Powles has treated some 400 patients in this manner over 18 years. In June 2000 the Marsden's prospective database contained 327 living myeloma patients, of whom the 14 were a part.[108] Barlogie certainly has some ten-year survivors but they are not mentioned in his studies which focus on improved overall and event-free survival in 1000 patients, in a 10-year span, for the lucky few with the right prognostic factors.

For we are indeed talking about a minority, though the statistics are complex. Both Barlogie and Powles focus on subgroups. Barlogie starts with 1000 patients and then finds that of 112 with the right prognostic factors, 52% achieve 5 years continuous complete remission. If we put the 112 back into the 1000 patients pool, 5.8% achieve CCR at 5 years. Powles, who has treated 400 patients with the new approaches, has 14 patients alive at the end of 10 years; 2 of these in continued remission at 15 and 16 years, with a median survival age of 11.6+ years. If we turn these 14 into a survivor percentage of the 400 treated, we get 3.5%. As a percentage of the 327 living myeloma patients recruited by the Marsden between April 1979 and May 2000, the 14 equal 4.3%.[108] This is not a very significant difference from the Mayo Clinic's 3% 10-year survival twenty years earlier.

The Mayo Clinic Study cited in our introduction was done in the pre-HDT therapy era. Most of the patients would have been treated with the standard Melphalan and/or radiation. Of these 570 (we have to exclude the 273 pre-chemo era patients) 3% were alive at 10 years. The comparable pre-HDT era, Barts 1992 survival curve for 156 unselected patients, already cited, has 4% alive at 10 years. (But, unlike the Mayo study, by the end of the first quarter of year 11 there are 0% survivors on the Barts curve.) Powles himself has noted the baffling phenomenon of relapse in Myeloma even after a continuous first remission beyond 10 years, not seen in other blood cancers such as acute leukaemia,[108] an enigma that remains to be deciphered if cure in Myeloma is to become a possibility. One has to conclude that though median survival may have improved with the new approaches, long-term survival remains elusive.

Now let us put the patient in a wider historical context: reported long-term survival in the standard therapy era, post-1964 and pre-1989, or thereabouts. (Of course, the new approaches were already underway in the 80s, but not yet widely available.) A review of the literature[108] reveals only 50 documented cases of survival beyond 10 years, with one patient reaching a record 31 years, and 12 others exceeding ten years, only two of whom made 20 years. Of these 50 patients, 8 died of cancers other than Myeloma. Melphalan is known to be carcinogenic. Only 4 patients out of the 50 are cited as "untreated." Long-term survival in Myeloma begins to look a little equivocal. Moreover it is clearly still a rare phenomenon. These 50 reported survivors are 50 out of literally hundreds of thousands of Myeloma cases worldwide in over 30 years.

Our patient has yet to cross the 10-year threshold. The decimal point has still to shift two places, from 0.5% to 0.005%. He is only 8 years out. But he is 8 years out "untreated." This in itself is even more remarkable. As we have seen, most long-term survivors to date have been treated, whether with standard chemo or the newer approaches. Not only has the patient achieved a more than comparable survival to the best that modern medicine has to offer, he has done this by following the ancient Hippocratic precept: "Primum non nocere." The same cannot be said of the medical approaches just discussed, which can have a mortality rate of anywhere between 15% up to 41%, if we include allogeneic bone marrow transplants.[110] If you choose to follow such a course of treatment, you risk your life to save your life, and often, the gamble fails. Or perhaps you just risk your life.

Of course, it cannot be said either that there are no risks in the patient's chosen course of treatment. It is, after all, an experiment, still ongoing, and life itself carries the risk of death, particularly for males the wrong side of 60. But given the risks and difficulties posed by still incurable Myeloma, perhaps this experiment merits some serious attention. The patient's continued survival does not look like chance. The odds at the beginning were too low for that to be the most indubitably obvious explanation. But then again, perhaps it is just luck, a statistical fluke. Is it necessary to wait another 12 years to establish this? The patient, at any rate, is not prepared to abandon any of his therapies just yet.

Only time and further research with Myeloma patients prepared to follow such "eccentric" protocols may finally settle this question. Such research is badly needed. Only perhaps something completely left of field will solve the enigma of Myeloma, and lead to real cures. New ideas are scarce in the clinical world of Myeloma. What conventional medical studies of Myeloma survival have achieved so far is to establish the self-evident fact that chances of survival are improved if Myeloma is diagnosed at a relatively early stage, with low β_2 microglobulin and CRP and absence of chromosome 13 deletion, and if patients respond well to treatment.[105] This does not go far enough: it is almost just description after the event. The questions to answer are *why* do certain patients respond better to treatment than others? What is biochemically different about them? *What* leads to such difference? *Why* are CRP, and β_2 microglobulin down? *What* keeps chromosome 13 stable *prior* to treatment? Case histories such as this may provide real clues. As St. Augustine once said, "Miracles do not happen in contradiction to Nature, only in opposition to what we *know* about Nature." The miraculous should heighten curiosity and investigation, not be dismissed as just a miracle.

Let me conclude with the biochemist, Dr. Jeffrey Bland: "Nutritional consultation should be a standard for every cancer therapy. In the face of our existing knowledge of the powerful convergence between the molecular biological origins of cancer and molecular nutrition, not to assess and treat every cancer patient nutritionally is a form of malpractice by omission."[111]

It is sincerely to be hoped that Michael will ultimately reach his goal, and beyond.

AFTERWORD

While it deals largely with Myeloma, the details of this Case History may be of real interest to all other cancer patients, particularly in the context of the patient's narrative history and his discussion of the role of temperament, a more scientifically elusive factor in cancer treatment.

I would like to offer this Case History as Case I, in a Best Case Series. By itself this Case History proves nothing. It is only an exalted and well documented anecdote. Anecdotes, however, if attended to, have frequently been the basis of good science. The National Cancer Institute has recently recognised this in the institution of its Best Case Series. Six such anecdotes, equally well documented, are all that is needed by the NCI to form the basis for further trials and investigations. Such a scheme not only recognises that good science is fed by anecdote, it is a major concession to the economic handicaps faced by underfunded and undersupported Complementary and Alternative Medicine, in the struggle to sift unproved from unprovable and gain acceptance by a conservative medical establishment. Thus if there are any Myeloma patients who feel strongly that they do not want to follow the conventional routes of chemotherapy and bone marrow transplants, but wish, on their own responsibility, and with the backing of their physicians, to follow the patient's protocols, I would advise that full medical records and details of treatment are kept. (It is also possible to *combine* some or all of the therapies discussed in the Case History with standard medical approaches to Myeloma. This approach may well reduce the risks of medical therapy and further enhance survival.) Orthomolecular Oncology, a registered UK and overseas charity, which is pioneering a special study of Myeloma, will be very pleased to hear from you. If you visit our website you may also enrol in a related, but less arduous, study, which also applies to MGUS patients. (Theoretically, this related study should remove the 25% risk of MGUS proceeding to Myeloma.) Our website contains a Patient's Resource Guide which should enable you to do most of the things described in this book. Please note, however, that your doctor and/or oncologist should play a central role at all times. Neither I nor Orthomolecular Oncology can take any legal responsibility for a patient's failure to use the considerable best that modern medicine has to offer. Nor do we advise against this.

Michael Gearin-Tosh: Medical Records

The medical data referred to throughout the Case History is available on the Orthomolecular Oncology website. Assuming the patient continues to survive, the complete records will be regularly updated, and hard copies can also be requested from the charity at any time. By the time of this book's publication a much needed, up to date and more fulsome bone marrow aspirate, including a plasma cell labelling index, cytogenetic investigation and thorough histology, should have been done. The results once more will be published on the website. If there is anything to be demonstrated finally by this Case History, such as that, at the very least, the patient's unorthodox therapies may have prevented disease progression, even without remission, this test should be reasonably definitive and provide more answers. My own speculation is that the patient may then be shown as having reverted to MGUS or the pre-Myeloma cancer stage. This would be achievement enough. The patient's only hesitation in doing the BMA test to date, apart from a busy working life, is that, feeling so well, he has been reluctant to submit to what he deems a form of torture, though doctors will gainsay this. There is also the understandable human fear of a return or progression of Myeloma. Science, however, demands sacrifices.

CORRESPONDENCE

To: Dr. Carmen Wheatley, D.Phil
(For Caliban Scripts Ltd)
Orthomolecular Oncology
The Estate Office
Ashton
Peterborough
PE8 5LE
UK

E-mail: canceraction@gtonline.net
Website: http://www.canceraction.org.gg

THANKS

To Michelle Levrier, Assistant Director of Orthomolecular Oncology, for help in collating all Michael's medical records.

ORTHOMOLECULAR ONCOLOGY

The charity, Orthomolecular Oncology, a registered cancer charity, was founded in 1999 (as a result of my experience in helping Michael) with the primarily educational aim of helping to disseminate internationally knowledge of the research and clinical work done with Adjuvant Nutritional Therapies in cancer, largely, but by no means exclusively, in North America. The scientific knowledge accumulating is impressive. Yet, paradoxically, it suffers from a major communication gap. It is almost as if there were a glass wall between scientists, on the one hand, and oncologists and physicians on the other. Yet, while we wait for the wonder cures of tomorrow, we could be implementing this knowledge in more integrated treatment now, with possibly enhanced outcomes, as Michael has done. Orthomolecular Oncology is a young and poor charity, but we have a great aim, which we hope can save many lives today. If you wish to learn more about our work (which includes fundraising for a scientific film, with BBC involvement, on the adjuvant nutrition in cancer movement in North America), or if you wish to help us in any way, we would be deeply grateful to hear from you. Alternatively, details, business plans, etc., can be supplied on request, or you may visit our website.

REFERENCES

1. Malpas J. S., Clinical Presentation and Diagnosis; Bergsagel D. E., Chemotherapy of Myeloma. Malpas J. S., Bergsagel D. E., Kyle R, Anderson K (eds). *Myeloma: Biology and Management,* Oxford University Press, 1998; 190; 294
2. Hoffbrand A. V., *Essential Haematology,* Oxford, 2001; p 328
3. Souhami R., Tobias J., Myeloma and other paraproteinaemias. *Cancer and Its Management,* Blackwell Science Ltd, 1998; 470–82
4. Malpas J. S. et al., op. cit.; 190
5. Kyle R. A., Long-term survival in Multiple Myeloma. *New Eng J of Med,* 1983; 308 (6): 314–16
6. Attal M., Harousseau J. L. et al., A prospective randomized trial of autologous bone-marrow transplantation and chemotherapy in multiple myeloma. *New Eng J of Med,* 1996; 335: 91–7
7. Ludwig H., Cohen A. M. et al., Interferon-alpha for induction and maintenance in multiple myeloma: Results of two multicenter randomized trials and summary of other studies. *Annals of Oncology,* 1995; 6: 467–76
8. Berenson S., Lichtenstein A. et al., Efficacy of pamidronate in reducing skeletal events in patients with advanced multiple myeloma. *New Eng J of Med,* 1996; 334: 488–93
9. Singhal S., Mehta J. et al., Antitumor activity of Thalidomide in refractory multiple myeloma. *New Eng J of Med,* 1999; 341 (21): 1565–71
10. Bergsagel P. L., Kuehl W. M., Molecular biology of multiple myeloma; Malpas J. S. et al., op. cit.: 48–69

11. Klein B., Zhang X. G., Rossi J. F., Cytokines, cytokine receptors and signal transduction in multiple myeloma. Malpas J. S. et al., op. cit.: 70–88

12. Personal communication to author in letter, dated 25 March 2000, from Dr. Christian Caritt, 137 Gloucester Road, London SW7 4TH

13. Malpas J. S., Clinical presentation and diagnosis. Malpas J. S., et al., op. cit.: 187–209

14. Bladé J., Kyle R., Monoclonal gammopathies of undetermined significance. Malpas J. S., et al., op. cit.: 513–44

15. Barth R., Frisch B., Bone marrow biopsy and aspiration for diagnosis of multiple myeloma. Malpas J. S. et al., op. cit.: 89–121

16. Personal communication to patient and the author by Dr. Tim Littlewood, Haematology Dept., John Radcliffe, Oxford.

17. Herrinton L. J., Weiss N. S., Olshan A. F., Epidemiology of Myeloma. Malpas J. S. et al., op. cit.: 150–86, 188

18. Gerson M., A Cancer Therapy. Gerson Institute, 1990, 81

19. Hildenbrand G., et al., Five year survival rates of melanoma patients treated by diet therapy after the manner of Gerson: a retrospective review. Alt The. Health Med, 1995; 1 (4): 29–37

20. Hildenbrand G., et al. The role of follow-up and retrospective data analysis in alternative cancer management: the Gerson Experience. J Neuropath Med, 6 (1): 49–56

21. Heber D., Blackburn G. L., Go V. L. W. (eds), Nutritional Oncology, Academic Press, San Diego, CA, 1999; 632. (Currently the key textbook.)

22. Hoffer A., Pauling L., Hardin Jones biostatistical analysis of mortality data for a second set of cohorts of cancer patients with a large fraction surviving at the termination of the study and a comparison of survival times of cancer patients receiving large regular oral doses of Vitamin C and other nutrients with similar patients not receiving these doses. J of Orthomolecular Med, 1993; 8 (3): 157–67

23. Pauling L., Cancer. How to Live Longer and Feel Better, New York, 1986, 217–42

24. Quillin P., Williams R. M.(eds), Adjuvant Nutrition in Cancer, Arlington Heights, IL, 1993, 380

25. Diamond J. W., Cowden W. L., Goldberg B., *Definitive Guide to Cancer,* Tiburon, CA, 1997: 1116
26. Sporn M. B., Roberts A. B., Goodman (eds), *The Retinoids, Biology, Chemistry and Medicine,* New York, 1994: 679
27. Quillin P., *Beating Cancer with Nutrition,* Tulsa, OK, 1998: 286
28. Jacobs M., *Vitamins and Minerals in the Prevention and Treatment of Cancer,* Boca Raton, FL, 1991
29. Simone C. B., *Cancer and Nutrition,* New York, 1992
30. Regular scientific international conferences that cover orthomolecular/nutritional oncology include: ISOM's Nutritional Medicine Today, annually at Toronto/Vancouver; Cancer Treatment Research Fund's Adjuvant Nutrition in Cancer Symposia; International Conference on Human Functioning, Wichita, KS; International CoEnzyme Q10 Association; The Danish Society of Orthomolecular Medicine's Health-Trends conferences; The World Conference series on Nutrition and Vitamin Therapy; the International Agency for Research on Cancer's European Conference on Nutrition and Cancer; NCI and NIH's Comprehensive Cancer Care Conferences, etc.
31. Green S., A critique of the rationale for cancer treatment with coffee enemas and diet; Lechner P., Hildenbrand G., Reply to Saul Green's Critique; JAMA vs. Gerson. *Townsend Letter for Doctors,* 1994; 5: 522–30
32. Bishop B., *A Time to Heal,* Arkana, 1996: 336
33. Cooke R., *Dr. Folkman's War: Angiogenesis and the Struggle to Defeat Cancer,* Random House, 2001: 365
34. Ulrich A., Chemotherapy of advanced epithelial cancer: a critical review. *Biomedicine and Pharmacotherapy,* 1992; 46: 439–52
35. Bailar J. C., Gormick H. L., Cancer Undefeated. *New Eng J of Med,* 1997; 336: 1569–74
36. Parkin D. M., Pisani P., Ferlay J., Global Cancer Statistics, *CA Cancer J Clin,* 1999; 49: 33–64
37. Malpas J. S., et al., op. cit.: 195
38. Tisdale M. J., New cachexic factors. *Current Opinion in Clinical Nutrition and Metabolic Care,* 1998; 1 (3): 253–6
39. Bougnoux P., n-3 Polyunsaturated fatty acids and cancer. *Current Opinion in Clinical Nutrition and Metabolic Care,* 1999; 2 (2): 121–6

40. Jiang W. G., Bryce R. P., Horrobin D. F., Essential fatty acids: molecular and cellular basis of their anti-cancer action and clinical implications. *Crit Rev Oncol Haematol,* 1998; 27: 179–209

41. Rose D. P., Connolly J. M., Rayburn J., Coleman M., Influence of diets containing eicosapentaenoic acid or docosahexaenoic acid on growth and metastasis of breast cancer cells in nude mice. *J of Nat Cancer Inst,* 1995; 87: 587–92

42. Bagga D., Capone S., et al., Dietary modulation of omega-3/omega-6 fatty acid ratios in patients with breast cancer. *J of Nat Cancer Inst,* 1997; 89: 1123–31

43. Koide T., et al., Antitumour effect of hydrolyzed anthocyanin from grape rinds and red rice. *Cancer Biotherapy and Radiopharmaceuticals,* 1996; 11 (4): 273–7

44. Middleton E. et al., Anticancer and Anticarcinogenic properties of plant flavonoids. Quillin P. (ed), *Adjuvant Nutrition in Cancer,* Arlington Heights, IL, 1994: 319–30

45. Stavric B., Quercetin in our diet: from potent mutagen to probable anticarcinogen. *Clin Biochem,* 1994; 27 (4): 245–8

46. Boon C. W., Kellof J. G., Cancer Chemoprevention. Heber et al. (eds), *Nutritional Oncology,* San Diego CA, 1999: 343–57

47. Pinto J. T., Rivlin R. S., Garlic and other allium vegetables in cancer prevention. Heber et al. (eds), op. cit.: 393–403

48. Combs G. F., Clark C. L., Selenium and Cancer. Heber et al. (eds), op. cit.: 215–222

49. Jang M. et al., Cancer chemopreventive activity of resveratrol, a natural product derived from grapes. *Science,* 1997; Jan. 10, 275 (5297): 218–20

50. Schwartz J. L., The clinical control of tumor cell growth through the action of carotenoids, retinoids and tocopherols. Quillin P. (ed), *Adjuvant Nutrition in Cancer,* Arlington Heights, IL, 1994: 173–233

51. Prasad K. N., Vitamin E induces differentiation and growth inhibition, and enhances the efficacy of therapeutic agents on cancer cells. Quillin P. (ed), op. cit.: 235–52

52. Zhang L. X. et al., Carotenoids enhance gap junctional communication and inhibit lipid peroxidation in C3H/10T1/2 cells: relationship to their cancer chemopreventive action. *Carcinogenesis,* Nov 1991; 12 (11): 2109–14.

53. Jansson B., Dietary, total body and intracellular potassium-to-sodium ratios and their influence on cancer. *Cancer Detection and Prevention,* 1990; 14 (5): 563–5
54. Kutsky R., Iodine. *Handbook of Vitamins, Minerals and Hormones,* New York, 1981: 138–
55. Shoden R. J., Griffin S., Iodine. *Fundamentals of Clinical Nutrition,* New York, 1980: 97
56. Kjellen E. et al., A therapeutic benefit from combining normabaric carbogen or oxygen with nicotinamide in fractionated X-ray treatments. *Radiotherapy Oncology,* Oct 1991; 22 (2): 81–91
57. Devlin T. M. (ed), *Textbook of Biochemistry with Clinical Correlations,* New York, 1997: 1186
58. Torosian M. H., Metabolic Abnormalities and Conditionally Essential Nutrients in the Cancer Patient. Quillin P. (ed), op. cit.: 157–172
59. Finke R. G., Coenzyme B_{12}-based chemical precedent for Co-C bond homolysis and other key elementary steps. Kraulter B. et al. (eds), *European Symposium on B12 and B12 Proteins,* 1998: 383–402
60. Savage D. G., Lindenbaum J., Folate-Cobalamin Interactions. Bailey L. B. (ed), *Folate in Health and Disease,* New York, 1995: 237–85
61. Lam K. T. et al., Isolation and identification of Kahweol palmitate and cafestol palmitate as active constituents in green coffee beans that enhance glutathione S-transferase activity in the mouse. *Cancer Res,* 1982; 42: 1193–8
62. Hirshberg C., Barasch M. I., *Remarkable Recovery,* BCA, 1995: 393
63. Foster H. D., Lifestyle influences on spontaneous cancer regression. *Int J Biosocial Res,* 1988; 10 (1): 17–20
64. Braverman E. R., *The Healing Nutrients Within, Facts, Findings and New Research on Amino Acids,* New Canaan, CT, 1997: 532
65. Pauling L., Cameron E., *Cancer and Vitamin C,* Philadelphia, 1993: 278
66. Klenner F. R., Significance of high daily intake of Ascorbic Acid in Preventive Medicine. Williams R. J., Kalita D. K. (eds), *A Physician's Handbook on Orthomolecular Medicine,* Keats Publishing Inc., 1977: 51–9, 207

67. Ogino T. et al., Oxidant stress and host oxidant defense mechanisms. Heber G. et al. (eds), op. cit.: 253–75
68. Hattersley J. G., CoEnzyme Q10 and Cancer. *J of Ortho Med,* 1996; 11 (1): 111–12.
69. Namba H., Maitake-D fraction: Healing and Preventive Potential for Cancer. *J of Ortho Med,* 1997; 12 (1): 43–9
70. European Aspirin Foundation, Aspirin in pain—the peripheral effects. *Aspirin Abstracts,* no. 14
71. Stephan J. et al., Increase by 10% of spine bone mineral density and effect on bone markers of 3-monthly intravenous injections of Ibandronate in osteoporosis in men with Klinefelter's Syndrome. *J of Bone and Mineral Research,* 2000; 15 (1): 226–
72. Schürch M. A. et al., Protein supplements increase serum insulin-like Growth Factor-1 levels and attenuate proximal femur bone loss in patients with recent hip fracture. *Annals of Int Med.,* 1998; 128 (110): 801–9
73. Petterson T. et al., Phosphate binding by a myeloma protein. *Acta Medica Scandinavica,* 1987; 222: 89–91
74. Sonnenblick M. et al., Paraprotein interference with colorimetry of phosphate in serum of some patients with multiple myeloma. *Clinical Chemistry,* 1986; 32: 1537–9
75. Head K., Ipriflavone: an important bone-building isoflavone. *Alternative Medicine Review,* 1999; 5 (1): 10–22
76. Larrick J. W., Therapeutic enzymes for cancer. Quillin P., (ed), op. cit.: 253–66
77. Ransberger K. et al., Medizinische Enzymforschungsgesellschaft. International Cancer Congress, Houston, 1970
78. Maurer H. R. et al., Bromelain induces the differentiation of leukemic cells in vitro: an explanation for its cytostatic effects? *Planta Med,* Oct 1988; 54 (5): 377–81
79. Solomon G. F., Emotions, Immunity and Disease. Temoshok et al. (eds), *Emotion in Health and Illness,* New York, 1983
80. Ader R., Felten D. I., Cohen N. (eds), *Psychoneuroimmunology,* San Diego, Academic Press, 1991
81. Pert C., Dienstfrey H., The neuropeptide network. *Annals of New York Academy of Sciences,* 1988; 521: 189–94
82. Pert C., *The Molecules of Emotion,* New York, 1997: 368

83. Gordon J. S., Curtin S., *Comprehensive Cancer Care,* New York, 2000: 314
84. Simonton C. O., Simonton S. M., Creighton J. L., *Getting Well Again,* Bantam Books, 1994
85. Anon., L-asparaginase in cancer therap., *Nutrition Reviews,* 1970; 28 (8): 206–9
86. Riordan N. H., Riordan H. D., et al., Intravenous ascorbate as a tumour cytoxic chemotherapeutic agent. *Med Hypothesis,* 1995; 44: 207–13
87. Jackson J. A., Riordan H. D., et al, High dose intravenous vitamin C and long time survival of a patient with cancer of the head of the pancreas. *J of Ortho Med,* 1995, 10 (2): 87–88
88. Hursting S. O. et al., Nutritional modulation of the carcinogenesis process. Heber G. et al. (eds), op. cit.: 91–104
89. Weindruch R. et al., *Hematol Oncol Clin North Am,* 1991; 5: 79–80
90. Vacca A. et al., Bone Marrow neovascularization, plasma cell angiogenic potential, and matrix metalloproteinase-2 secretion parallel progression of human multiple myeloma. *Blood,* 1999; 93 (9): 3064–73
91. Weissman I. L., Cooper M. D., How the immune system develops. *Life, Death and the Immune System; Scientific American*: special issue, New York, 1994: 136
92. Mason J. B., Levesque T., Folate: effects on carcinogenesis and the potential for cancer chemoprevention. *Oncology,* 1996; 10 (11): 1727–43
93. Pauling L., The Immune System; Pauling L., op. cit., 128–36
94. Park C. H., Kimler B. F., Growth modulation of human leukaemic, preleukemic and myeloma progenitor cells by L-ascorbic acid. *Am J Clin Nutr,* 1991; 54: 1241 S-465
95. Phillips E. J. et al., Infections in myeloma. Malpas J. S. et al. (eds), op. cit.: 439–76
96. Hallek K. et al., Multiple myeloma: increasing evidence for a multistep transformation process. *Blood,* 1998; 91 (1): 3–21
97. Lawson-Matthew P. et al., Vitamin D metabolism in Myeloma. *British J of Haematology,* 1989; 73: 57–60

98. De Luca H. F., New concepts of Vitamin D function. *Ann NY Acad Sci,* 1992; 669: 59–69

99. Klein B. et al., Murine anti-interleukin-6 monoclonal antibody therapy for a patient with plasma cell leukaemia. *Blood,* 1991; 78: 1198–1204

100. Bataille R. et al., Biologic effects of anti-interleukin-6 murine monoclonal antibody in advanced multiple myeloma. *Blood,* 1995; 86: 685–91

101. Sato K. et al., Reshaping a human antibody to inhibit the interleukin-6 dependent tumour cell growth. *Cancer Research,* 1993; 53: 851–56

102. Sporeno E. et al., Human IL-6 receptor super agonists with high potency and wide spectrum on multiple myeloma. *Blood,* 1996; 87: 4510–19

103. Berger L. C., et al., Interferon-beta interrupts interleukin-6 dependent signalling events in myeloma cells. *Blood,* 1997; 89 (1): 261–71

104. Anthes J. C. et al., Interferon-alpha down-regulates the interleukin-6 receptor in a human multiple myeloma cell line U266. *Biochem J,* 1995 (Pt 1); 309: 175–80.

105. Osgood E. E., The survival time of patients with plasmocytic myeloma. *Cancer Chemotherapy Reports,* 1960; 9: 1–10

106. Barlogie B., High-Dose therapy and innovative approaches to treatment of multiple myeloma. *Seminars in Hematology,* 2001; 38 (2) suppl 3: 21–7

107. Sirohli B., Powles R. et al., Complete remission rate and outcome after intensive treatment of 177 patients with IgG Myeloma. *British J of Haematology,* 1999; 107: 656–66

108. Powles R., personal communication to author re total number of Myeloma patients treated in 18 years. Powles R., Sirotin B. et al., Continued first complete remission in Multiple Myeloma for over 10 years: a series of "operationally cured" patients. Abstracts of the 42nd Annual Meeting of the American Society of Hematology, 1–5 December 2000, San Francisco, CA, 132

109. Rosner F. et al., Ten-year survival in multiple myeloma: Report of two cases and a review of the literature. *New York State J of Med,* 1992; 2 (7): 316–18

110. Gharton G. et al., An overview of allogeneic transplantation in multiple myeloma. Program and abstracts of the

VIII International Myeloma Workshop; 4–8 May 2001; Banff, Alberta, Canada. Abstract S14

111. Bland J., Lecture given at the 1995 Adjuvant Nutrition in Cancer Treatment Symposium, Tampa, FL

BIBLIOGRAPHY
TO *LIVING PROOF*
AND *WHY LIVING PROOF?*

Jennifer Barraclough, ed., *Integrated Cancer Care,* Oxford, 2001

Beata Bishop, *A Time To Heal,* London, 1985

Max Black, *Language and Philosophy: Studies in Method,* Cornell, 1949

George Blackburn, David Heber and Vay Liang W. Go, *Nutritional Oncology,* San Diego, 1999

William Boyd, *The Spontaneous Regression of Cancer,* Illinois, 1966

Simon Carr, *The Boys Are Back in Town,* London, 2001

Anton Chekhov, *Lady with Lapdog and Other Stories,* translated by David Magarshack, Harmondsworth, 1964

Anton Chekhov, *Letters of Anton Chekhov,* edited by Simon Karlinsky, New York, 1973

Peter J. D'Adamo, *Eat Right for Your Type,* New York, 1996

J. de Vries, *Cancer and Leukaemia,* Edinburgh, 1988

Cornélie de Wassenaer, *A Visit to St. Petersburg 1824–5,* translated by Igor Vinogradoff, Norwich, 1994

John Diamond, *C: Because Cowards Get Cancer Too,* London, 1998

John Donne, *Sermons,* ed. G. R. Potter and E. M. Simpson, Berkeley, 1953

Max Gerson, *A Cancer Therapy,* New York, 1958 (fifth edition 1990)

Mel Greaves, *Cancer: The Evolutionary Legacy,* Oxford, 2000

Halifax: Complete Works, edited by J. P. Kenyon, London, 1969

Václav Havel, *Letters to Olga,* 1983, translated by Paul Wilson, London, 1990

Hippocrates, *Of Ancient Medicine* and *Precepts*

C. Hirshberg and M. I. Barasch, *Remarkable Recovery,* New York, 1995

B. K. S. Iyengar, *Light on Yoga,* London, 1966 (1991 edition)

Jacques Jouanna, *Hippocrate* (1992), translated by M. B. DeBevoise, Baltimore, 1999

John Keats, *Letters,* ed. H. E. Rollins, Cambridge, 1958

Lesley Kenton, *Raw Energy,* London, 1994

James Le Fanu, *The Rise and Fall of Modern Medicine,* London, 1999

Primo Levi, *If This Is a Man,* London, 1979

Russian Journal of Lady Londonderry 1836-7, edited by W. A. L. Seaman and J. R. Sewell, London, 1973

Bryan Magee, *Confessions of a Philosopher,* London, 1997

James G. Malpas, Daniel E. Bergsagel, Robert Kyle and Ken Anderson, *Myeloma: Biology and Management,* Oxford 1998 (second edition)

John Mann, *The Elusive Magic Bullet,* Oxford, 1999

P. B. Medawar, *The Future of Man,* Oxford, 1960

Arthur Miller, *Timebends,* London, 1987

Candace Pert, *Molecules of Emotion,* New York, 1997

Ruth Picardie, *Before I Say Goodbye,* Harmondsworth, 1998

Jane Plant, *Your Life in Your Hands,* London, 2000

Roy Porter, *The Greatest Benefit to Mankind,* London, 1997

G. J. G. Rees, S. E. Goodman and J. A. Bullimore, *Cancer in Practice,* Oxford, 1993

Jean Renoir, *Renoir My Father,* translated by R. and D. Weaver, London, 1962

Helen Rollason, *Life's Too Short,* London, 2000

Peter Selby, *Confronting Cancer,* London, 1993

Dmitri Shostakovich, *Memoirs,* edited by Solomon Volkov, London, 1979

Aleksandr Solzhenitsyn, *Cancer Ward,* translated by Nicholas Bethell and David Burg, Harmondsworth, 1971

Anne Somerset, *Elizabeth I,* London, 1991

Robert Souhami and Jeffrey Tobias, *Cancer and Its Management,* London, 1998

Liz Tilberis, *No Time to Die,* London, 1998
Lewis Thomas, *The Medusa and the Snail,* New York, 1974
Lewis Thomas, *The Youngest Science,* New York, 1983
Mary Warnock, *A Memoir: People and Places,* London, 2000
David Weatherall, *Science and the Quiet Art,* Oxford, 1995
Robert Weinberg, *One Renegade Cell,* London, 1998
Geoffrey R. Weiss, *Clinical Oncology,* Connecticut, 1993
W. B. Yeats, *Essays and Introductions,* London, 1961

ACKNOWLEDGMENTS

I have written this book at the suggestion of Sir James Gowans FRS.

Henry Dale Research Professor of the Royal Society, 1962–77, and Secretary of the Medical Research Council in Britain, 1977–87, James has been a Fellow of St. Catherine's, also my college in Oxford, since 1961. Throughout my illness he has been ready to comment on doctors and on perspectives of my own, and he has guided my reading.

My manuscript has been read by Sir James and also by Dr. Christian Carritt, Professor Robert A. Kyle of the Mayo Clinic, Rochester, Minnesota, USA, Professor Ray Powles of the Royal Marsden Hospital, London, and Professor Sir David Weatherall FRS of Oxford University.

Benjamin Ross has encouraged me at all stages, as has David Ambrose, who has also given me the benefit of his practical acumen. I am fortunate to have Ian Chapman as my publisher.

People who have played a major part in my experience of cancer have confirmed, where possible, my recollections.

I am also grateful for suggestions from Helen Gummer, my U.K. editor, Beth Wareham, my U.S. editor, and from Laurence Ambrose, Arkadius, Aby Bidwell, Simon Bowes Lyon, Michael Codron, Christopher Darbyshire, Anne

Denham, Fram Dinshaw, Dr. Godfrey Fowler, Katia Hadidian and her family, Sergei and Natasha Issayev, Drue Heinz, Tessa Keswick, Dr. Veronica Lyell, Dr. Nina Kobiashvili, Dr. Dmitry Myrney, John Morrison, Raymond Plant, Olga Polizzi, Diana Rigg, Dr. Hugh Riordan, Ronny Schwartz, Patrick Sergeant, J. C. Smith and Anthony Storr.

Rufus Waddington has been a sounding board for ideas and he rescued my disc from computer damage.

Carmen Wheatley has helped me beyond the events of my history, and this book is dedicated to her with thanks.